To my mother and father
and in memory of my grandmother

The publishers would like to thank Rosemary Steele and the Agfa Gevaert copyproof process for the Kirlian text and photographs on pp. 64 and 65, Hardlines for the drawing on p. 66, Jennie Brown for the drawings on pp. 7 and 8, Helen Reed for all the plant drawings and Roddy Paine for the commissioned photographs.

British Library Cataloguing in Publication Data

Brown, Denise
  Aromatherapy. – (Headway Lifeguides
  Series)
  I. Title II. Series
  615

  ISBN 0–340–55950–0

First published 1993

© 1993

Typeset by Wearset, Boldon, Tyne and Wear
Printed in Great Britain for the educational publishing division of Hodder & Stoughton Ltd, Mill Road, Dunton Green, Sevenoaks, Kent by Thomson Litho Ltd

HEADWAY LIFEGUIDES

AROMATHERAPY

Headway · Hodder & Stoughton

CONTENTS

INTRODUCTION

The value of Aromatherapy

Aromatherapy is a truly holistic therapy which uses essential oils in treatments to strive for physical, mental and spiritual health equilibrium. The body's innate ability to heal itself is awakened and gentle persuasion encourages a return from a state of imbalance or 'dis-ease' to a state of balance or health. This healing process occurs irrespective of whether the disharmony is manifesting itself on a seemingly physical level (for example a headache) or on an emotional level (for example depression).

Aromatherapy is not only aimed at relieving and eliminating health problems but is also very much concerned with the prevention of disease and the promotion of healthy living. Essential oils allow us to raise our levels of resistance and immunity to disease. Serious health problems are not given the chance to develop and you can feel happier, healthier, fitter and full of life!

Many hundreds of thousands of lay people are now using essential oils successfully on themselves and their families in the home. This book provides a simple and informative introduction to Aromatherapy and will enable you to use them *safely* and *effectively* as part of your daily life. Although essential oils may offer a gentle and natural alternative to many drugs when treating for common ailments, I must emphasise the necessity to consult your doctor where problems are persistent or serious.

Another word of warning! Aromatherapy is very addictive and once exposed to these powerful, therapeutic essences they will become part of your life evoking within you a deep probing desire to learn more and more about the fascinating art of Aromatherapy. As I sit here writing this book I am surrounded by the wonderful and inviting fragrances of my essential oils – my source of inspiration. Follow me into this alluring world of Aromatherapy and explore this ancient therapeutic art. Life will never be quite the same again!

A brief history of Aromatherapy

The healing powers of aromatic oils have been harnessed for thousands of years. The ancient Egyptians imported plant materials from distant lands employing them for a multitude of purposes. They used them in magical and religious ceremonies as offerings to honour their deities.

The dead were anointed and embalmed in preparation for the after-life. The infamous incense *Kyphi* was formulated and applied as a perfume and taken as a medicine to soothe and dispel anxieties and fears.

In the Bible there are numerous references to the use of oils for healing and religious purposes. We are all well aware that two of the gifts brought by the Three Kings were frankincense and myrrh. Both essential oils are highly regarded and prized today.

Historians relate that during the Middle Ages the perfumers enjoyed an immunity to cholera and other life-threatening diseases. Oils normally employed to hide the unpleasant smells of unwashed bodies were used as a form of protection and to fight epidemics and infections.

Unfortunately with the rapid progress of scientific knowledge during the nineteenth century, oils were replaced by chemical ingredients. These synthetic copies, although effective as perfumes, did not impart the same therapeutic value and they very often resulted in extremely unpleasant side-effects.

Fortunately essential oils were rediscovered by the French chemist, Professor René M. Gattefosse who coined the term aromatherapy in 1928. After severely burning his hand one day in a laboratory experiment he plunged it into the nearest container of liquid which happened to be lavender essence. To his astonishment the pain was relieved and the burns healed rapidly leaving no trace of a scar. This led him into experimentation with essential oils and he discovered that they greatly accelerated the healing process.

His important work was developed by the renowned Dr Jean Valnet. His famous book *The Practice of Aromatherapy* is regarded by many to be the 'Bible of Aromatherapy'.

Nowadays the use of pure essential oils is growing in popularity across the world as a means of alleviating symptoms and promoting good health. Confronted with the complications and side-effects of orthodox drugs, people are now turning to natural medicines for both relief and protection.

1
ESSENTIAL OILS

What are essential oils?

Essential oils are natural aromatic liquid substances often considered to be the 'life force', the 'soul' or the 'hormones' of plants. These essences are capable of inducing a state of harmony and well-being in body, mind and spirit and they promote and maintain health. Every essential oil is endowed with its own particular therapeutic properties. All aromatic essences are extremely powerful antiseptics capable of destroying bacteria and viruses. The immune system may be stimulated raising the resistance of the body to disease. Growth of new cells may be encouraged, thus delaying the process of ageing by eliminating old cells more quickly. Circulation may be improved, pain relieved, fluid retention reduced, nerves are calmed and much more.

Essential oils, unlike many other substances, are able to penetrate through the skin due to their small molecules. They may then be absorbed into the bloodstream and into the lymphatic system. Natural organic aromatic essences are extremely safe, when used properly, and they have the advantage over drugs in that they leave no toxic residues behind since they are excreted by the body. The side-effects are virtually non-existent.

Methods of extraction

Distillation
This is by far the most widely used method.

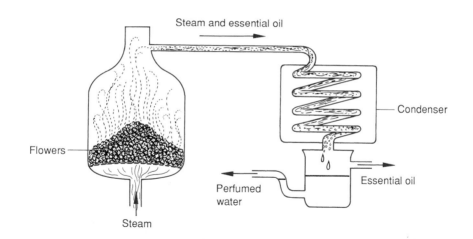

The plant is heated with water or steam or both in a still and the vapour is then channelled through a condenser. The emerging liquid is a mixture of oil and water and since essential oils are not water soluble they can be easily separated from the water. Depending on the essence, a heavy oil will sink beneath the water whereas a lighter oil will float on the surface. The water travelling round the distillation plant becomes impregnated with perfume and is useful as perfumed water such as rose or lavender water.

Enfleurage

This method is sometimes employed for the extraction of essential oils from delicate flowers such as jasmine and involves the use of purified cold fat which is spread over sheets of glass mounted in large rectangular wooden frames. Flowers are strewn upon this layer of fat which absorbs the essential oil. After approximately a day the flowers are removed and replaced by fresh ones. This process is repeated many times until the fat is saturated with the oil. The saturated fat is washed in alcohol and then carefully heated. Since alcohol evaporates first the pure essential oil remains. Obviously this method is very time-consuming and labour-intensive and the aromatic substances produced by this method are extremely expensive. Vast quantities of flowers are required to produce

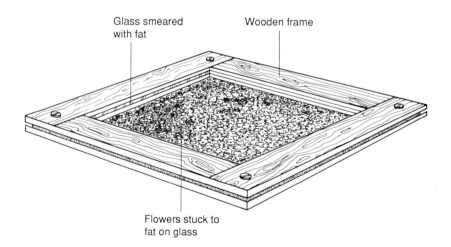

Glass smeared with fat
Wooden frame
Flowers stuck to fat on glass

just a small amount of oil. For example, 2,000 kilograms of jasmine petals yield just one kilogram of essential oil and 30 roses are required to produce just one drop!

Maceration

This process is very similar to enfleurage but involves the use of hot rather than cold fat. The flowers are placed into hot oil until their cells rupture causing the absorption of the essential oil. The flowers are strained off, and the process repeated until the oil is saturated with perfume. It is then treated as for enfleurage.

Solvent extraction

The flowers of plants are covered with a solvent which extracts the aromatic substance. This is then filtered and the solvent is evaporated so that the essential oil remains. This process may be used for gums, resins and flowers.

Expression

This process is employed for the extraction of oil from the citrus family such as orange, lemon, bergamot and tangerine. The peel is squeezed and the oil is collected in a sponge which, when saturated, is squeezed out. This method was formerly performed by hand but is now, unfortunately, often performed by machine to cut down the cost.

Base oils

Pure essential oils are usually far too highly concentrated to be used either undiluted or directly on the skin. They must be used with great care in the correctly diluted dosage since any excess could be harmful.

It is important to choose a pure, good quality vegetable oil to act as a carrier for your essential oils. Mineral oil (usually referred to as baby oil) is a very unsuitable medium because of its very low penetration power which restricts the essential oil from passing through the skin. In fact, it is far more beneficial to massage babies with a pure vegetable oil than with baby oil, which is lacking in nutrients and is not easily absorbed.

There are a vast number of vegetable, nut and seed oils to choose from and it is an advantage that many vegetable oils possess therapeutic properties themselves. Sweet almond, grapeseed, soya bean, olive, sunflower, safflower, corn and hazelnut are all good general base oils. Grapeseed oil is one of the least expensive and fortunately has no smell. Other vegetable oils may be added to the general base oil to increase penetration: small amounts of nourishing avocado or peach kernel oil will benefit dry skin. Wheatgerm is also a good carrier oil for mature or dehydrated skin and is useful to add since it helps to preserve the oil. Jojoba oil, although expensive, is my particular favourite, especially for the face. It helps to alleviate dry, inflamed skin, psoriasis, eczema and acne

Care and storage

Essential oils are highly volatile, which means that they evaporate very quickly, and are damaged by ultraviolet light and extremes of temperature. Therefore they should be stored in amber coloured glass bottles and should not be decanted into clear glass or plastic bottles. Any oils sold in clear glass bottles cannot possibly be pure essential oils and are of no benefit. Always keep your oils at an even temperature – neither too hot nor too cold – and ensure that the tops are tightly closed when they are not in use.

Pure essential oils will last for approximately one to two years but once diluted in a carrier oil they have a shelf life of only about three months.

It is vital to choose only *pure* essential oils in order to benefit from aromatherapy. Synthetic oils may have a pleasant smell but they simply do not possess therapeutic properties – they will not work. Take care not to buy essential oils that have already been diluted in a carrier oil and are being sold as pure essential oils. Do not be deterred by the cost. Although true essential oils are expensive such small amounts are used that the cost is actually minimal.

2

AROMATHERAPY TREATMENT TECHNIQUES

There are a whole host of ways to enjoy and derive benefit from essential oils. I will outline some of the easiest and most effective techniques of application.

Massage and blending

Massage is merely an extension of our fundamental instinctive need to touch and to be touched. A child will run to its mother's arms to have a sore knee rubbed better or to have the pain of a stomach ache eased. A grieving adult will find great comfort and solace in the caring arms of another. Massage even *without* essential oils is a very powerful tool. (Refer to my other book in this series on *Massage*.) Pure essential oils and massage coupled together are even more powerful. Massage is undoubtedly the most effective and beneficial method of application and the art of aromatherapy massage is discussed in detail in this book. The aromatic oil is quickly absorbed by the skin and taken into the bloodstream.

Essential oils must be blended with a suitable carrier oil in the appropriate dilution. When blending essential oils and base oils it is important to bear in mind that an increased concentration of essential oil does *not* imply that the therapeutic formula will be more effective. A 2 to 3 per cent dilution is desirable to avoid unpleasant side-effects and reactions. Since a teaspoon holds approximately 5 ml, I suggest that you use only 3 to 4 drops of pure essential oil to 2 teaspoons of base oil. Although it is difficult to believe, you will only require a few teaspoons of oil in your aromatherapy massage.

When blending, consider both the physical complaints and emotional problems of the recipient of the treatment. It is vital to consider their emotional state since many physical ailments stem from an emotional source. I strongly recommend the selection of at least one oil for any emotional imbalances. You are treating the whole person, not the symptoms, searching for the root cause.

Be creative with your blending and always remember the golden rule – if you like the aroma it is doing you good. We are instinctively drawn to the essential oils which are right for us at the time. It is vital to allow the recipient to smell the aromatic formula before applying it since the effects of the aromatherapy treatment will be completely ruined if the aroma is not pleasurable.

Facial oils

When blending a facial oil the percentage of essential oil to carrier oil is less than for a body oil. Use a ½ to 2 per cent dilution.

Normal skin

Add 2 to 3 drops of essential oil to every 10 ml (two teaspoons) of carrier oil.

Sensitive skin

Add 1 drop of essential oil to every 10 ml of carrier oil gradually increasing the dosage.

The following formulae are per 50 ml of carrier oil since you will probably prefer to mix a larger quantity rather than blending your mixture daily.

- For a *normal skin* add 15 drops of pure essential oil.

- For a *sensitive skin* add 5 drops of pure essential oil, gradually increasing the dosage to 10 drops if no sensitivity is apparent.

Choose two or three essential oils for your blend making a total of 15 drops.

Acne/oily skin
Bergamot
Cypress
Geranium
Juniper
Lavender
Lemon
Lemongrass
Neroli
Sandalwood
Tea-tree

Example
6 drops bergamot
4 drops geranium
5 drops cypress

= 15 drops to 50 ml base oil

Dry skin
Chamomile
Geranium
Jasmine
Lavender
Neroli
Rose
Sandalwood

Example
5 drops geranium
2 drops rose
8 drops sandalwood

= 15 drops to 50 ml base oil

Mature, ageing, wrinkles
Clary sage
Frankincense
Myrrh
Neroli
Rose
Sandalwood

Example
4 drops frankincense
8 drops lavender
3 drops neroli

= 15 drops to 50 ml

Normal skin
Frankincense
Geranium
Jasmine
Lavender
Neroli
Rose

Example
5 drops geranium
8 drops lavender
2 drops rose

= 15 drops to 50 ml

Sensitive skin
Chamomile
Lavender
Neroli
Rose

Example
6 drops lavender
1 drop neroli
1 drop rose

= 8 drops to 50 ml

Please note that when blending I use fewer drops of the heavier, more powerful, costly oils.

For specific skin conditions such as dermatitis, eczema, psoriasis, etc. please refer to the therapeutic index on page 52.

Ointments and creams

Ointments

To prepare an ointment you will need:

- Yellow beeswax

- Sweet almond oil (or avocado, jojoba, etc.)

Use one part of beeswax to four parts of oil e.g.

- 10 gm yellow beeswax

- 40 ml almond oil

Place the beeswax and almond oil in a heat-proof dish in a pan of hot water. Melt over a gentle heat stirring continually until the mixture has melted. Remove from the heat and allow to cool.

Add 15 drops of pure essential oil(s) of your choice. Put the cream into *amber* coloured pots and store in a cool place.

Facial/hand creams

Very often people will prefer to apply a cream to the face and hands rather than an oil. They are under the mistaken apprehension that an oil will give the skin a shiny appearance. You will need:

- 10 gm yellow beeswax

- 40 ml almond oil (or any other vegetable oil)

- 20 ml distilled water (or lavender water, orange water or rose water)

Melt the beeswax and almond oil in one bowl in a pan of water over a gentle heat. Heat the distilled water in another bowl over a gentle heat to blood temperature (37°C). Remove from the heat. Add the warm distilled water *gradually* to the oil mixture beating all the time.

Add 15 drops of the essential oil(s) of your choice. Put the cream into *amber* coloured jars and store in a cool place.

Baths

Aromatherapy baths have been employed for pleasure and therapeutic purposes throughout history. Hippocrates, the father of medicine, claimed that 'the way to health is to have an aromatic bath and a scented massage every day.' Baths were particularly enjoyed by the ancient Egyptians who had public baths, as did the Romans for whom they were an important aspect of social life. Water itself is very therapeutic and 'water cures' are advocated by naturopaths, and various forms of hydrotherapy can be found in use nowadays at health farms and natural therapy centres. Water and aromatic oils provide a powerful combination having synergistic effects.

Essential oils are very simple to use in the bath. Just fill the bath and scatter about 6 drops of your chosen undiluted essential oil into the water, agitating thoroughly. Do not add the essential oil until you have run the bath completely, otherwise the oil will evaporate with the heat of the water and the therapeutic properties will be lost before you climb in! Always disperse the oil – if you inadvertently sat down on neat essential oil of, say tangerine, you would jump up again very quickly! Shut the door to keep the precious aromas in and stay in the bath for at least 15 minutes to allow the oil to penetrate deeply into the tissues.

If you so desire, you may blend your 6 drops of essential oil with a couple of teaspoons of carrier oil. This is particularly beneficial for those with dry skin. Choose any vegetable oil such as sweet almond, wheatgerm, avocado or jojoba. You could mix up enough oil for several baths. Your skin will feel soft, nourished and supple.

I would strongly advise those of you with a sensitive skin *always* to blend the essential oil with a carrier oil. When using essential oils in a bath for babies and young children they should also be diluted. Undiluted essential oils can damage the eyes and babies and toddlers do have a tendency to rub their eyes. Use just 1 drop in the baby's bath and 2 drops in a toddler's bath. I can wholeheartedly support the effectiveness of this method.

Any essential oil may be added to the bath. Please exercise caution with the citrus oils and the stronger essences such as **black pepper** and **peppermint** if you have particularly sensitive skin. Just add 3 drops instead of 6.

All conditions may be treated employing aromatic bathing and recipes will be given throughout the book. However, here are a few suggestions to start you off as you are probably dying to try them out! You may choose a single oil or a combination of oils remembering not to use more than a **total** of 6 drops.

As you plunge yourself deeply into your aromatherapy bath, relax and enjoy the healing powers of the essential oils. As a general rule if you like the aroma, it is doing you good.

Relaxing to promote sleep and relieve tension
Roman chamomile (my favourite, rather costly but well worth the expense!), **lavender, marjoram, sandalwood.**

Stimulating and invigorating to wake you up
Black pepper, lemon, peppermint, rosemary.

Aches and pains
Black pepper, chamomile, frankincense, juniper, lavender, marjoram, thyme.

Fluid retention
Cypress, fennel, juniper, lemon.

Aphrodisiac
Jasmine, rose, sandalwood, ylang ylang.

Coughs and colds
Cajeput, eucalyptus, tea-tree, thyme.

Immune system booster
Chamomile, lavender, tea-tree, thyme.

Footbaths and handbaths

Footbaths and handbaths are highly beneficial in situations where it is impractical to enjoy a full aromatherapy bath – perhaps if you are elderly or have a disability. Footbaths, in particular, are incredibly relaxing at the end of a long, hard day.

Add about 6 drops of essential oil to a bowl of hand hot water just before you immerse the feet and soak for about 10 to 15 minutes.

Sitz baths

A sitz bath is invaluable in cases of cystitis, haemorrhoids, vaginal discharges, itching and so on. Sprinkle about 6 drops of pure essential oil into a bowl of hand hot water and sit in the bowl for about 10 minutes.

Compresses

Compresses can be used for a variety of disorders such as muscular aches and pains, bruises, rheumatic and arthritic pain, headaches and sprains.

Compresses may be applied either hot or cold. Alternate hot and cold compresses are invaluable for sprains. As a general rule, where there is fever, acute pain or hot swellings, use a cold compress. When treating chronic (i.e. long-term) pain use a hot compress.

To make a compress mix approximately 6 drops of essential oil into a *small* bowl of water. Soak any piece of absorbent material such as a flannel, piece of sheeting or towelling in the solution ensuring that as much essential oil as possible is absorbed onto your fabric. Squeeze out the compress so it is not dripping everywhere and apply to the affected area. Wrap clingfilm around it or secure with a bandage. Leave for about two hours or even overnight. Where there is fever replace with a new compress when necessary.

Inhalations

Inhalations are particularly beneficial for respiratory problems such as colds, sinusitis, sore throats, catarrh, colds and so on.

Although you may think that the simplest method is to open the bottle of essential oil and inhale, this is not a good idea. Firstly, frequent opening of essential oils accelerates the rate of evaporation and therapeutic properties are lost, and secondly spilling 2 ml of say pure essential oil of rose on your carpet would be very costly!

Add approximately 4 drops of pure essential oil to a bowl of hot water. Cover the head with a towel and lean over the bowl inhaling deeply for about five minutes. Keep eyes closed to avoid irritation.

Caution: Asthmatics should not use this method as concentrated steam may induce an attack.

Essential oils may also be inhaled by placing a few drops on a handkerchief: use 2 drops of **eucalyptus** if you have sinusitis or a cold. A couple of drops of an appropriate oil such as **chamomile** or **lavender** may be scattered onto the pillow to relieve insomnia.

Diffusers and room fresheners

Electronic diffusers known as nebulisers are useful since essential oils may pass into the atmosphere without being heated and thus altered. Nebulisers are now becoming popular in hospitals and if you can afford one they are very valuable in the home. To use, just place a few drops of essential oil into the nebuliser and switch it on.

It is also possible to purchase a small clay burner. These are readily available. Put a few teaspoons of water in the loose bowl on the top and sprinkle approximately 6 drops of essential oil into it. Light the nightlight and the oils will diffuse into the air.

Alternatively simply place 6 drops of your chosen pure undiluted oil into any small bowl of boiling water. Place the bowl in a warm place.

A few drops of essential oil may also be sprinkled onto a small cotton wool ball and placed in warm strategic places such as on a radiator. You may also use a simple small plant spray filled with water to which you have added approximately 10 drops of oil.

Whichever method you choose make sure that you shut the door to derive maximum benefit. Use oils such as **lavender** and **chamomile** to create an atmosphere of relaxation and to calm any 'up-tight' friends! Enliven the atmosphere with essential oils of **lemon** or **tangerine**. Banish those germs with **tea-tree**, **lavender**, **lemon** and **thyme**. Unblock sinuses and lungs with **eucalyptus** and **cajeput**. Stimulate the brain with **basil** and **rosemary**. There are so many exciting possibilities.

Internally

Although *pure* essential oils may be taken internally I would strongly advise against this method of treatment unless it is strictly supervised.

Essential oils are approximately 50 to 100 times more powerful than the herbs from which they are derived. A herb may be quite safe whereas an essential oil is hazardous and ingestion of oils can have serious or even fatal consequences. The methods of external application which I have described are all highly effective and they do not directly involve the participation of the digestive system. When the oils come into contact with the chemical contents of the stomach their chemistry is radically altered.

FOR SAFETY'S SAKE PLEASE *DO NOT TAKE BY MOUTH*.

Contraindications

As a general rule most essential oils are safe provided they are used properly and sensibly. However, please observe the following at all times:

- Do not take internally.

- Do not apply essential oils to the skin undiluted (except for **lavender** and **tea-tree** for first aid purposes) as they are far too concentrated and can result in inflammation and allergic reaction.

- Do not get the oils into the eyes.

- Keep the oils out of reach of young children.

- Ensure that the dosage is accurate as too much essential oil can be harmful.

- Purchase only *pure* essential oils.

- Take care with particularly sensitive skins – it is possible to do a patch test if you are anxious. (See appendix for oils likely to cause sensitivity.)

- Do not massage where there is a high fever. The body has already raised itself to a high temperature to fight off the infection and does not need the burden of even more toxins to deal with. However, essential oils may be applied on compresses in order to reduce temperature.

- Do not massage the abdomen heavily during pregnancy and especially for the first three months where risk of miscarriage is at its highest. Beware of certain oils throughout pregnancy. (See appendix.)

- Beware of infectious skin conditions.

- Use only very light pressure over severe varicose veins.

- Beware of *recent* scar tissue, open wounds and areas of inflammation.

- Always dilute essential oils when adding them to a baby's or child's bath.

- Avoid exposure to strong sunshine or sunbeds immediately *after* an aromatherapy massage.

- Wait a couple of hours after a sauna since the pores are open as the body is still eliminating.

PLEASE REFER TO THE LIST OF HAZARDOUS ESSENTIAL OILS IN THE APPENDIX.

3

THIRTY ESSENTIAL OILS A–Z

There are in fact, several hundred essential oils but I have listed the most common oils including many of my own personal favourites.

Perhaps this list of essential oils may seem overwhelming at first but with practice and experience you will easily and rapidly find the information you need.

The lists of properties and indications are by no means exhaustive but I have listed the most important benefits.

For simplification I have included my **Keywords** which indicate at a glance the main effects of each oil. The system of classification into top, middle or base notes refers to their volatility – the rate of evaporation. Top notes are highly volatile, evaporating most rapidly, whereas base notes evaporate more slowly. Base notes will, in fact, 'fix' other essences i.e. they will slow down the evaporation rate of the top and middle notes. Usually top notes will uplift and stimulate, middle notes will balance and base notes will calm and sedate.

Any precautions that must be observed are listed at the end of each essential oil under **Contraindications**. Suggestions for blending are also included although you needn't adhere to these combinations rigidly. Be creative and adventurous! Why not begin your collection with just five or six essential oils? Then buy one oil a month. Remember, be guided by your aroma preference since the body instinctively knows what its requirements are.

Basil

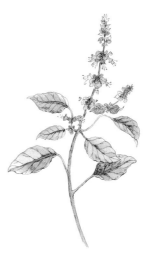

Latin name	*Ocimum basilicum*
Family	*Labiatae*
Note	Top
Essence from	Whole plant of herb
Fragrance	Pleasant, aniseed-like, minty

Principal properties and indications

Keywords

- Uplifting,
- Strengthening
- Clarifying
- Stimulating
- Decongestive

Digestive
Use in bath, compress, diffuser, inhalation, massage

- Difficult and painful digestion
- Gastric spasm
- Intestinal infections
- Vomiting

Head
Use in bath, compress, diffuser, inhalation, massage

- Catarrh
- Earache
- Fainting and vertigo
- Headache and migraine
- Nasal polyps
- Rhinitis
- Sinusitis

Neurological/emotional
Use in bath, diffuser, inhalation, massage

- **Basil** is an excellent nerve tonic. It first stimulates and then calms the person down
- Anxiety and depression
- Inability to concentrate
- Indecision
- Mental fatigue
- Nervous tension

Respiratory
Use in bath, compress, diffuser, inhalation, massage

- Asthma
- Bronchitis
- Colds and coughs
- Emphysema
- Hiccoughs
- Whooping cough

Miscellaneous

- Insect repellent – especially wasps and mosquitoes

Contraindications

1 Use in low dilution to avoid skin irritation

2 Avoid during pregnancy

3 High doses can be stupefying

Blends well with bergamot, geranium

Benzoin

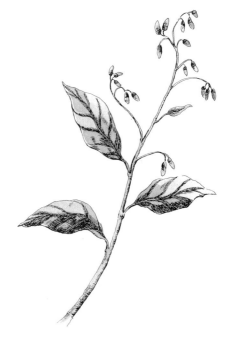

Latin name	*Styrax benzoin*
Family	*Styraceae*
Note	Base
Essence from	Gum of tree trunk
Fragrance	Heavy, liqueur-like, warm

Principal properties and indications

Keywords
- Soothing
- Warming
- Gets things moving
- Comforting
- Healing

Circulatory
Use in bath, massage
- Poor circulation
- Heart tonic

Genito-urinary
Use in bath, compress, massage, sitz bath
- Cystitis
- Discharges
- Fluid retention
- Urinary infections

Neurological/emotional
Use in bath, diffuser, inhalation, massage
- Anxiety
- Grief
- Exhaustion (emotional, physical or psychic)
- Loneliness
- Sadness

Respiratory
Use in bath, compress, diffuser, inhalation, massage
- Asthma
- Bronchitis
- Colds, coughs, flu
- Laryngitis
- Throat infections

Skin care
- Cracked and chapped skin
- Dermatitis
- Redness
- Skin irritation
- Sores and wounds

Blends well with rose

Bergamot

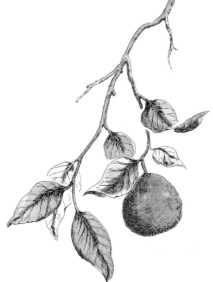

Latin name	*Citrus bergamia*
Family	*Rutaceae*
Note	Top
Essence from	Peel of fruit
Fragrance	Sweet, citrus, floral, refreshing

Principal properties and indications

Keywords
- Antidepressant
- Antiseptic
- Balancing
- Uplifting

Genito-urinary
Use in bath, massage, sitz bath

- Cystitis (relieves physical causes, emotional tension and depression)
- Discharges
- Urinary infections
- Vaginal pruritis (itching)

Neurological/emotional
Use in bath, diffuser, inhalation, massage

- Anxiety states – uplifting yet sedative
- Depression

Skin care
Use in bath, compress, massage

- Acne, oily skin
- Boils, carbuncles
- Chickenpox
- Eczema
- Greasy scalp
- Herpes
- Psoriasis

Contraindications

1 Do not use neat on the skin and do not apply before sunbathing as **bergamot** increases the photosensitivity of the skin. (Hence its inclusion in sun-tan preparations.)

2 Take care with sensitive skin

Blends well with almost all other oils

Black pepper

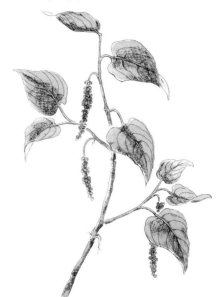

Latin name	Piper nigrum
Family	Piperacea
Note	Middle
Essence from	Berries
Fragrance	Spicy, hot, pungent

Principal properties and indications

Keywords
- Stimulant
- Tonic
- Warming
- Eliminative

Circulatory
Use in bath, compress, massage

- Anaemia
- Fever
- Poor circulation

Digestive
Use in bath, compress, diffuser, inhalation, massage

- Colic
- Constipation
- Food poisoning
- Flatulence
- Heartburn
- Loss of appetite

- Nausea and vomiting
- Stimulant

Muscular/joints
Use in bath, compress, massage
- Arthritis
- Muscular aches and pains
- Muscle stiffness
- Rheumatism
- Toothache

Neurological/emotional
Use in bath, compress, diffuser, inhalation, massage
- Coldness (use **black pepper** for physical and emotional coldness)
- Grief
- Impotence
- Neuralgia
- Stimulates
- Strengthens the nerves

Respiratory
Use in bath, compress, diffuser, inhalation, massage
- Catarrh
- Colds and coughs
- Flu
- Phlegm

Blends well with frankincense, rosemary

Cajeput

Latin name	Melaleuca leucodendron
Family	Myrtaceae
Note	Top
Essence from	Leaves and buds
Fragrance	Penetrating, eucalyptus-like

Principal properties and indications
Keywords
- Antiseptic
- Penetrating
- Stimulating
- Warming

Digestive
Use in bath, massage
- Diarrhoea
- Gastric spasm
- Indigestion

Muscular/joints
Use in bath, compress, massage
- Neuralgia
- Rheumatism

Respiratory
Use in bath, compress, diffuser, inhalation, massage
- Asthma
- Bronchitis
- Colds
- Laryngitis and throat infections
- Sinusitis

Contraindications
Take care with sensitive skin

Blends well with lavender

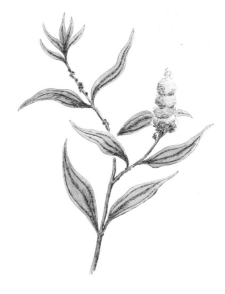

Chamomile

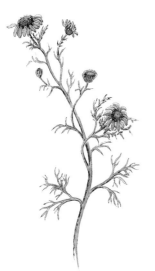

Latin name	*Anthemis nobilis* (Roman Chamomile) *Matricaria chamomilla* (German Chamomile)
Family	*Compositae*
Note	Middle
Essence from	Flowers of the plant
Fragrance	Apple-like, light, aromatic, sharp

Principal properties and indications

Keywords
- Balancing
- Calming
- Soothing
- Children

Roman chamomile is an excellent remedy for use with infants – very similar to **lavender**. It is low in toxicity and can be used for all children's complaints – colic, ear and throat infections, irritability, temper tantrums, skin infections, allergies and asthma. It contains azulene which is an excellent anti-inflammatory agent which, although not present in the fresh flower, is formed when the plant is distilled.

Circulatory
Use in compress, diffuser, inhalation, massage

- Anaemia
- Stimulates the white blood cells (leucocytes) and therefore boosts the immune system
- Fevers (encourages sweating and combats fever)

Digestive
Use in bath, compress, diffuser, inhalation, massage

- *All* digestive problems and in particular children's digestive problems (colic, stomach pains, diarrhoea)
- Colitis
- Difficult and painful digestion
- Flatulence
- Liver and spleen congestion
- Vomiting

Genito-urinary
Use in bath, compress, massage, sitz bath

- *All* female disorders, especially when associated with nervous tension
- Particularly indicated for menopause, PMT, painful or irregular periods, scanty or absent menstruation, excessive blood loss
- Diuretic
- Vulvar itching

Head
Use in bath, compress, diffuser, inhalation, massage

- Earache
- Headaches and migraine
- Neuralgia
- Teething pains/ toothache/ gingivitis

Muscular/joints
Use in bath, compress, massage

- All aches and pains whether in the muscles, joints or organs
- Cramp and stitch
- Dull aches
- Muscular aches
- Rheumatism

Neurological/emotional
Use in bath, compress, diffuser, inhalation, massage

- Depression
- Hysteria
- Insomnia
- Irritability, restlessness, impatience, states of anger, oversensitivity

Skin care
Use in bath, compress, massage

- Acne
- Allergies (eruptions due to allergies e.g. urticaria)
- Burns
- Dry, inflamed skin
- Enlarged capillaries
- Sensitive skin

Blends well with geranium, lavender, rose

Clary sage

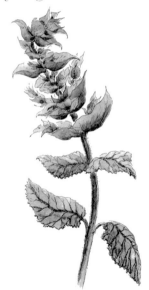

Latin name	Salvia sclarea
Family	Labiatae
Note	Top/middle
Essence from	Flowering tops
Fragrance	Strong, sweet, heady, floral, slightly musky

Principal properties and indications

Keywords

- Euphoric, intoxicating, sedative, tonic, **clary sage** is used by many aromatherapists in preference to **sage** as it is considered to be safer

Genito-urinary
Use in bath, compress, massage

- Childbirth. It encourages the contractions but aids relaxation
- PMT
- Painful menstrual cramps
- Scanty menstruation
- Tonic for the womb – balances the female reproductive system

Neurological/emotional
Use in bath, diffuser, inhalation, massage

- Frigidity and impotence
- Nervous exhaustion and general debility (physical, mental, nervous, sexual)
- Stress and tension

Skin care
Use in bath, compress, massage

- Particularly useful for soothing and cooling inflammation
- Aged skin, wrinkles
- Dry skin
- Oily skin (and scalp)
- Sunburn

Contraindications

1 Avoid during pregnancy

2 Do not take alcohol and **clary sage** together as this may lead to headaches and nightmares

Blends well with bergamot, geranium, juniper, lavender, rose, sandalwood

Cypress

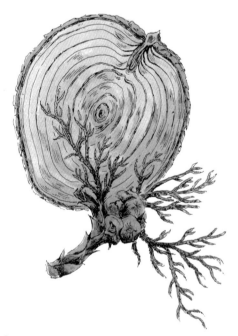

Latin name	Cupressus sempervirens
Family	Coniferae

Note	Middle
Essence from	Twigs and branches
Fragrance	Woody, balsamic

Principal properties and indications

Keywords
- Astringent,
- fluid reducing,
- warming and reviving,
- tonic

Circulatory
Use in bath, compress, massage, sitz bath
- Haemorrhoids
- Poor circulation
- Varicose veins

Genito-urinary
Use in bath, compress, massage
- Fluid retention
- Heavy and painful periods
- Incontinence of urine (enuresis)
- Menopause
- PMT

Neurological/emotional
Use in bath, diffuser, inhalation, massage
- Irritability and nervous tension
- Strengthening and comforting – eases grief and is useful in times of change

Respiratory
Use in bath, compress, diffuser, inhalation, massage
- Asthma
- Cough
- Whooping cough

Skin care
- Broken capillaries
- Cellulite
- Excessive perspiration (especially of the feet) – reduces both sweating and odour
- Varicose veins

Blends well with bergamot, clary sage, juniper, lavender, neroli

Eucalyptus

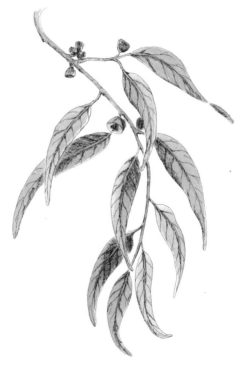

Latin name	*Eucalyptus globulus*
Family	*Myrtaceae*
Note	Top
Essence from	Leaves of tree
Fragrance	Fresh, camphor-like

Principal properties and indications

Keywords
- Antiseptic
- Expectorant
- Stimulant

Circulatory
Use in bath, compress, diffuser, inhalation, massage
- Fever – cooling effect
- Infectious diseases – will prevent from spreading

Digestive
Use in bath, massage, sitz bath
- Diarrhoea
- Diabetes – helps to balance the blood sugar level
- Worms

Genito-urinary
Use in bath, compress, massage, sitz bath
- Cystitis
- Fluid retention
- Urinary infections

Muscular
Use in bath, compress, massage
- Arthritis
- Fibrositis
- Muscular and rheumatic pains
- Rheumatism

Neurological/emotional
Use in bath, diffuser, inhalation, massage
- Energy imbalance
- Exhaustion

Respiratory
Use in bath, compress, diffuser, inhalation, massage
- All respiratory disorders
- Asthma
- Bronchitis
- Catarrh, colds, cough
- Flu
- Sinusitis
- Throat infections

Skin care
Use in bath, massage
- Antiseptic – cuts
- Burns and scalds
- Herpes
- Measles and other infectious diseases

Miscellaneous
Use in diffuser
- Insect repellent

Blends well with bergamot, lavender

Fennel (sweet)

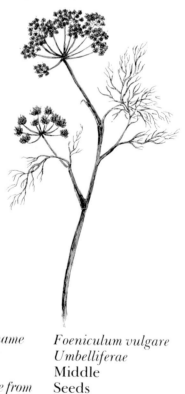

Latin name	Foeniculum vulgare
Family	Umbelliferae
Note	Middle
Essence from	Seeds
Fragrance	Aniseed-like, camphor-like, strong

Principal properties and indications

Keywords
- Detoxifying
- Digestive
- Eliminative
- Fluid reducing

Highly prized by the Greeks and Romans. Greek athletes ate fennel to give them strength without putting on weight. Roman women ate it to prevent weight gain and the men ate it to give energy

Digestive
Use in bath, compress, massage
- *All* digestive and intestinal problems
- Colic
- Constipation
- Digestive stimulant
- Flatulence
- Food poisoning
- Hiccoughs
- Nausea
- Obesity
- Stomach pains

Genito-urinary
Use in bath, compress, massage
- Fluid retention
- Insufficiency of milk in nursing mothers
- Kidney stones
- Menopausal irregularities
- Scanty menstruation
- Stimulates the body to produce its own oestrogen
- Toxic elimination

Neurological/emotional
Use in bath, compress, massage
- Alcoholism (reduces the effects of alcohol on the body)
- Anorexia

Respiratory
Use in bath, compress, massage
- Bronchitis
- Flu
- Shortness of breath

Skin care
Use in bath, compress, massage
- Cellulite
- Orange peel skin
- Toxic-congested skin

Contraindications

1 Fennel is not advisable for young children

2 Avoid during pregnancy

3 Excessively high doses can disturb the nervous system – avoid if you are epileptic.

Blends well with geranium, juniper, lavender, rose, sandalwood

Frankincense

Latin name	*Boswellia thurifera*
Family	*Burseraceae*
Note	Base
Essence from	Gum of the bark of tree
Fragrance	Balsamic, camphor-like, lingering, spicy, woody

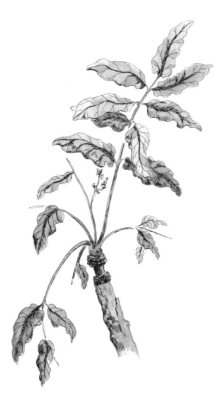

Respiratory
Use in bath, compress, diffuser, inhalation, massage

- *All* respiratory complaints – both physical and emotional benefits
- Asthma
- Bronchitis
- Catarrh
- Cough
- Lung disorders
- Slows down and deepens the breath

Skin care
Use in bath, compress, massage

- *All* skin care
- Prevents ageing – mature skin will rejuvenate
- Tonic effect – may help wrinkles
- Ulcers and wounds

Blends well with black pepper, geranium, lavender, sandalwood

Principal properties and indications
Keywords

- Cooling
- Comforting
- Decongestive
- Healing
- Elevating
- Expectorant
- Rejuvenating

One of my favourite oils!

Neurological/emotional
Use in bath, diffuser, inhalation, massage

- Elevating yet soothing effects on the emotions
- Enables those stuck in the past to move on
- Fears
- Grief
- Obsessions

Geranium

Latin name	Pelargonium odorantissimum
Family	Geraniaceae
Note	Middle
Essence from	Flowers, leaves and stalks
Fragrance	Sweet, strong, rose-like

Principal properties and indications
Keywords

- Antidepressant
- Balancing
- Fluid reducing

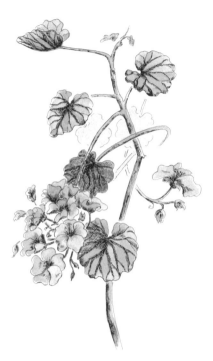

Respiratory
Use in bath, diffuser, inhalation, massage

- Sore throat
- Tonsillitis

Skin care
Use in bath, compress, massage

- *All* skin types – balancing
- Astringent
- Bleeding
- Bruises
- Burns, wounds, ulcers – very healing
- Dry eczema
- Inflamed, oily and combination skin

Miscellaneous
- Insect and mosquito repellent

Blends well with almost all oils especially the citrus oils (bergamot and geranium are an excellent combination) and rose

- Healing
- Uplifting

Digestive
Use in bath, massage

- Diabetes
- Diarrhoea
- Liver/gall bladder problems

Genito-urinary
Use in bath, compress, massage

- Fluid retention
- Kidney stones
- Menopause – it balances the hormones
- PMT
- Sterility

Neurological/emotional
Use in bath, compress, diffuser, inhalation, massage

- Anxiety states
- Depression
- Neuralgia

Ginger

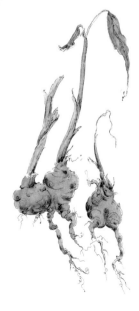

Latin name	Zingiber officinale
Family	Zingiberaceae
Note	Top
Essence from	Roots
Fragrance	Aromatic, hot, spicy, zingy

Principal properties and indications

Keywords
- Digestive
- Fiery
- Warming
- Stimulant

Circulation
Use in bath, compress, massage
- Fever
- Poor circulation

Digestive
Use in bath, compress, massage
- *All* digestive problems
- Diarrhoea
- Difficult digestion
- Flatulence
- Loss of appetite
- Nausea (travel sickness or early morning sickness)
- Stomach cramps

Muscular/joints
Use in bath, compress, massage
- Arthritis
- Muscular aches and pains
- Rheumatism
- Sprains

Neurological/emotional
Use in bath, diffuser, inhalation, massage
- Confidence
- Courage
- Poor memory

Respiratory
Use in bath, diffuser, inhalation, massage
- Catarrh
- Colds and flu
- Sore throat
- Tonsillitis

Contraindications
Use in low dilutions to avoid skin irritations

Blends well with juniper, lavender, rosemary, citrus oils

Jasmine – 'King of essential oils'

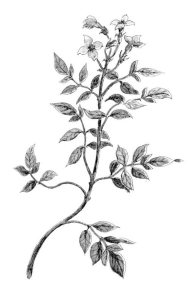

Latin name	Jasminum officinale
Family	Jasminaceae
Note	Base
Essence from	Flowers
Fragrance	Exhilarating, exotic, exquisite, floral, sweet, warming

Principal properties and indications

Keywords
- Antidepressant
- Aphrodisiac
- Euphoric
- Healing
- Uplifting

Genito-urinary
Use in bath, compress, massage
- Childbirth – relieves pain and promotes the birth. Helps to expel the placenta
- Frigidity and impotence – the best aphrodisiac releasing inhibition and strengthening the male sex organs
- Menopause
- Uterine disorders

Neurological/emotional
Use in bath, diffuser, inhalation, massage
- **Jasmine** is of great value in psychological and psychosomatic problems
- Anxiety
- Apathy
- Aphrodisiac
- Depression (even post-natal)
- Lack of confidence
- Lethargy
- Sadness
- Uplifting

Skin care
Use in bath, compress, diffuser, inhalation, massage
- *All* skin care
- Dermatitis
- Dry, sensitive skin

Blends well with geranium, neroli, rose, sandalwood citrus oils,

Juniper

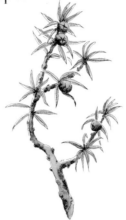

Latin name	*Juniperus communis*
Family	Coniferae
Note	Middle
Essence from	Berries or branches
Fragrance	Balsamic, hot, sharp

Principal properties and indications
Keywords
- Antiseptic
- Cleansing
- Detoxifying
- Fluid reducing
- Purifying
- Tonic

Circulatory
Use in bath, compress, massage, sitz bath
- Arteriosclerosis
- Fever
- Haemorrhoids

Digestive
Use in bath, compress, massage
- Diabetes
- Difficult digestion
- Flatulence
- Food poisoning
- Loss of appetite
- Sluggish digestion
- Tonic
- Worms

Genito-urinary
Use in bath, compress, massage

- Cystitis
- Difficulty in passing urine
- Discharges
- Enlarged prostate
- Fluid retention
- Low output of urine
- Kidney stones
- Painful menstruation
- Scanty menstruation
- Urinary infections

Muscular/joints
Use in bath, compress, massage

- Arthritis
- Gout
- Rheumatism

Neurological/emotional
Use in bath, diffuser, inhalation, massage

- Anxiety
- Depression
- Loss of memory
- Nervous exhaustion
- It is an excellent oil for times when you feel emotionally depleted. It clears waste from the mind just as it does from the body

Skin care
Use in bath, compress, massage

- *All* skin disorders
- Acne and oily skin
- Cellulite
- Dermatitis
- Eczema
- Ulcers and wounds
- *Skin conditions may get worse before they improve since* **juniper** *stimulates the body to throw off toxins*

Contraindications
Avoid during pregnancy (some say)

Blends well with bergamot, cypress, fennel, frankincense, lavender, sandalwood

Lavender

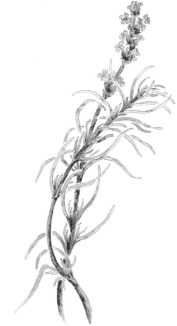

Latin name	Lavandula officinalis
Family	Labiatae
Note	Middle
Essence from	Flowering tops
Fragrance	Clean, flowery

Principal properties and indications

Keywords
- Antidepressant
- Antiseptic
- Balancing
- Calming
- Healing
- Rejuvenating

Lavender is probably the most precious of all the essential oils. It is so versatile that its properties are too numerous to mention

Circulatory
Use in bath, compress, diffuser, inhalation, massage
- Fevers – reduces fever and prevents the spread of infection
- Heart tonic
- High blood pressure
- Palpitations
- Stimulates the white blood cells and thus the immune system

Digestive
Use in bath, compress, massage
- *All* digestive disorders – especially in children
- Colic
- Diarrhoea
- Difficult and painful digestion
- Flatulence
- Nausea and vomiting
- Worms

Genito-urinary
Use in bath, compress, diffuser, inhalation, massage, sitz bath
- Childbirth – speeds up the delivery, calms the mother and purifies the air
- Cystitis
- Discharges
- Fluid retention
- Low output of urine
- PMT
- Menopause
- Menstrual pain
- Scanty menstruation

Head
Use in bath, compress, diffuser, inhalation, massage
- Alopecia and all types of baldness of nervous origin
- Bad breath
- Earache
- Fainting
- Headache and migraine
- Throat infections and laryngitis
- Vertigo

Muscular/joints
Use in bath, compress, massage
- *All* muscular aches and pains. Reduces pain and inflammation, relaxes, tones
- Arthritis
- Rheumatism
- Sprains

Neurological/emotional
Use in bath, compress, diffuser, inhalation, massage
- Anxiety

- Depression
- Insomnia
- Irritability
- Mental and physical debility
- Mood swings
- Panic and hysteria

Respiratory
Use in bath, compress, diffuser, inhalation, massage

- Asthma
- Bronchitis
- Catarrh
- Colds
- Coughs
- Flu
- Sinusitis
- Throat infection
- Whooping cough

Skin care
Use in bath, compress, massage

- *All* skin care – oily, dry, sensitive etc. It is anti-inflammatory, antiseptic, soothing and regenerates and rejuvenates the skin
- Acne
- Athlete's foot
- Boils
- Burns
- Carbuncles
- Dermatitis
- Eczema
- Mature, ageing skin
- Psoriasis
- Sensitive skin
- Sunstroke
- Ulcers
- Wounds and sores of all descriptions

Miscellaneous
Use in diffuser

- Insect bites and stings (use neat)

Blends well with almost all oils especially citrus oils, black pepper, clary sage, geranium, marjoram, neroli, rosemary

Lemon

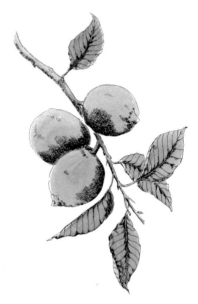

Latin name	*Citrus limonum*
Family	*Rutaceae*
Note	Top
Essence from	Rind of fruit
Fragrance	Clean, crisp, fruity, refreshing, sharp

Principal properties and indications
Keywords

- Alkaline
- Antiseptic
- Detoxifying
- Fluid reducing
- Purifying
- Stimulant
- Tonic

Circulatory
Use in bath, compress, diffuser, inhalation, massage

- Anaemia
- Arteriosclerosis
- Chilblains
- High blood pressure
- Liquifies the blood
- Poor circulation
- Stimulates white blood cells boosting the immune system
- Varicose veins

Digestive
Use in bath, compress, massage

- **Lemon** is an alkalising agent and a gastric antacid. To relieve hyperacidity drink a glass of water daily into which you have squeezed the juice of half a lemon
- Diarrhoea
- Flatulence
- Heartburn
- Hyperacidity of the stomach
- Liver congestion
- Obesity
- Stomach ulcers

Genito-urinary
Use in bath, compress, massage

- Fluid retention
- Kidney stones
- Thrush

Head
Use as a gargle (one or two drops to a glass of water)

- Gingivitis
- Laryngitis
- Mouth ulcers
- Tongue and mouth inflammation

Muscular/joints
Use in bath, compress, massage

- Arthritis
- Gout
- Rheumatism

Respiratory
Use in bath, compress, diffuser, inhalation, massage

- Asthma
- Bronchitis
- Catarrh
- Colds
- Flu
- Laryngitis and sore throats
- Lung infections
- Sinusitis

Skin care
Use in bath, compress, massage

- Cellulite – it stimulates the lymphatic system
- Eruptions and diseases of all kinds
- Boils
- Cuts and infected wounds
- Greasy skin
- Herpes
- Scabies
- Varicose veins
- Warts and verrucae (apply neat)

Miscellaneous
Use in diffuser
- Prevents the spread of diseases

Contraindications
Take care with sensitive skin and in sunlight

Blends well with cypress, frankincense, juniper, lavender, neroli

Lemongrass

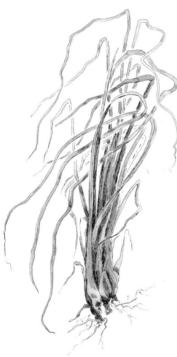

Latin name	Cymbopogon citratus
Family	Graminae
Note	Top
Essence from	Grass
Fragrance	Fresh and lemony

Principal properties and indications
Keywords
- Refreshing
- Tonic
- Astringent

Digestive
Use in bath, compress, massage
- Colic
- Colitis
- Difficult digestion
- Flatulence
- Loss of appetite

Genito-urinary
Use in bath, massage
- Fluid retention
- Promotes milk supply

Skin
Use in bath, massage, compress
- Acne
- Excessive sweating
- Open pores
- Scabies
- Tonic

Miscellaneous
Use in diffuser
- Insect repellent, prevents spread of infectious diseases

Contraindications
Take care with sensitive skin

Blends well with geranium, lavender

Marjoram (sweet)

Latin name	Origanum marjorana
Family	Labiatae
Note	Middle
Essence from	Flowering tops
Fragrance	Sweet, powerful, warming

Principal properties and indications
Keywords
- Calming
- Digestive

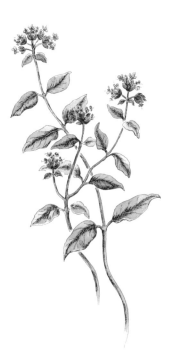

- Pain-relieving
- Sedative

Circulatory
Use in bath, massage
- High blood pressure
- Heart tonic

Digestive
Use in bath, compress, massage
- Colic
- Constipation
- Difficult and painful digestion
- Flatulence

Genito-urinary
Use in bath, compress, massage, sitz bath
- Excessive sexual impulses
- Irregular periods
- Painful periods
- PMT
- Vaginal discharges

Muscular/joints
Use in bath, compress, massage
- Arthritis
- Bruises
- Rheumatism
- Sprains and strains

Neurological/emotional
Use in bath, diffuser, inhalation, massage
- Anxiety
- Grief – comforting and warming
- Hysteria
- Insomnia
- Nervous tension

Respiratory
Use in bath, compress, diffuser, inhalation, massage
- Asthma
- Bronchitis
- Coughs and colds

Contraindications
Avoid during pregnancy

Blends well with bergamot, lavender, rosemary

Myrrh

Latin name	Commiphora myrrha
Family	Burseraceae
Note	Base
Essence from	Gum of the bark
Fragrance	Balsamic, musty

Principal properties and indications
Keywords
- Antiseptic
- Catarrh
- Healing
- Rejuvenating
- Soothing

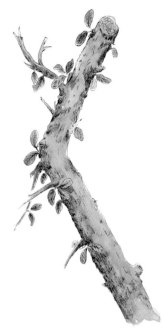

Genito-urinary
Use in bath, compress, massage, sitz bath

- Absence of menstruation
- Discharges
- Thrush
- Uterine disorders

Head
Use as a gargle (two drops to a glass of water)

- Gingivitis
- Mouth infections
- Mouth ulcers and inflammations
- Pyorrhoea
- Sore throats

Respiratory
Use in bath, compress, diffuser, inhalation, massage

- Asthma
- Bronchitis
- Catarrh
- Cough
- Hoarseness and loss of voice

Skin care
Use in bath, compress, massage

- Antiseptic, healing, anti-inflammatory and cooling
- Athlete's foot
- Cracked and chapped skin
- Inflamed skin
- Rejuvenating – ageing, mature, wrinkled skin
- Ulcers and wounds
- Weeping eczema

Contraindications
Avoid during pregnancy

Blends well with bergamot, lavender

Neroli

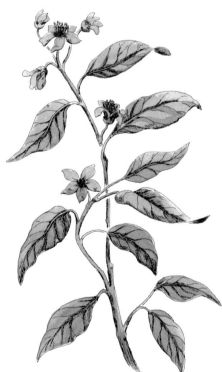

Latin name	*Citrus aurantium*
Family	*Rutaceae*
Note	Base
Essence from	Flowers
Fragrance	Floral, sweet, delicious

Principal properties and indications

Keywords
- Antidepressant
- Aphrodisiac
- Sedative
- Stress and tension

Circulatory
Use in bath, compress, diffuser, inhalation, massage
- Cardiac spasm and false angina
- Lowers high blood pressure
- Palpitations

Digestive
Use in bath, compress, diffuser, inhalation, massage
- Butterflies in stomach
- Diarrhoea (stress induced)
- Flatulence
- Nervous dyspepsia

Neurological/emotional
Use in bath, compress, diffuser, inhalation, massage
- One of the most effective sedative/antidepressant oils
- Anxiety – long term or short term (e.g. before an exam)
- Aphrodisiac
- Grief
- Hysteria and panic
- Insomnia
- Nervous tension
- Shock

Skin care
Use in bath, compress, massage
- *All* skin types – it is rejuvenative
- Broken veins
- Dry skin
- Irritation and redness
- Sensitive skin

Blends with almost all oils especially citrus oils, geranium, jasmine, rose and sandalwood

Patchouli

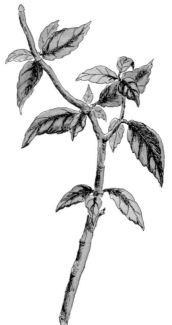

Latin name	*Pogostemon patchouli*
Family	*Labiatae*
Note	Base
Essence from	Leaves
Fragrance	Heavy, musty, strong

Principal properties and indications
Keywords
- Antidepressant
- Healing
- Rejuvenative
- Soothing
- Very popular oil in the Sixties

Neurological/emotional
Use in bath, diffuser, inhalation, massage

- **Patchouli** is stimulating in very small doses yet relaxing in larger doses
- Anxiety
- Aphrodisiac
- Confusion and indecision
- Depression
- Lethargy and sluggishness

Skin care
Use in bath, compress, massage

- Acne
- Allergies
- Cracked and chapped skin
- Dandruff
- Dermatitis
- Eczema
- Fungal infections e.g. athlete's foot
- Inflamed and red skin
- Rejuvenative – ageing, wrinkled skin
- Weeping sores

Blends well with bergamot, geranium, ginger, juniper, citrus oils

Peppermint

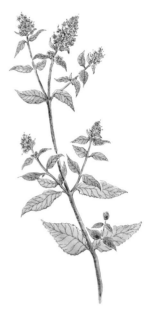

Latin name	Mentha piperita
Family	Labiatae
Note	Middle
Essence from	Leaves and flowering tops
Fragrance	Refreshing, reviving, sharp

Principal properties and indications
Keywords
- Cooling
- Digestive
- Pain relieving
- Stimulating
- Tonic

Circulatory
Use in bath, compress, massage

- Anaemia
- Fevers – induces sweating and cools down

Digestive
Use in bath, compress, massage

- *All* digestive problems
- Colic

- Diarrhoea
- Flatulence
- Indigestion
- Liver conditions
- Loss of appetite
- Nausea and vomiting – sea-sickness and travel-sickness
- Sluggish digestion
- Stomach pains

Genito-urinary
Use in bath, compress, massage

- Painful periods
- Scanty menstruation

Head
Use in bath, compress, massage

- Headaches and migraine – especially food related. It works well with **lavender**
- Sinus congestion and headache
- Toothache (1 drop neat on the affected tooth)

Muscular/joints
Use in bath, compress, massage

- All muscular and joint problems where pain relief is required

Neurological/emotional
Use in bath, compress, diffuser, inhalation, massage

- Clears the mind
- Impotence
- Mental and general fatigue
- Neuralgia
- Shock and hysteria

Respiratory
Use in bath, compress, diffuser, inhalation, massage

- Asthma – especially food related
- Bronchitis
- Colds
- Coughs
- Flu

Skin care
Use in bath, compress, massage

- It is cooling, anti-inflammatory and decongestive
- Acne
- Dermatitis
- Redness and irritation
- Scabies – good for infectious diseases
- Sunburn

Contraindications

1 Take care with sensitive skins

2 Store away from homoeopathic medicine

Blends well with lavender, marjoram, rosemary

Rose – 'Queen of essential oils'

Latin name	Rosa damascena
Family	Rosaceae
Note	Base
Essence from	Flowers, petals
Fragrance	Exquisite, heady, lingering, loving

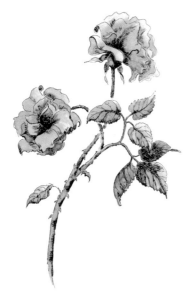

Principal properties and indications

Keywords
- Antidepressant
- Aphrodisiac
- Balancing
- Female problems
- Rejuvenating
- Uplifting

Possibly my favourite oil!

Circulatory
Use in bath, massage
- Cleanses the blood
- Tonic for the heart

Digestive
Use in bath, compress, massage
- Constipation
- Liver conditions
- Nausea

Genito-urinary
Use in bath, compress, diffuser, inhalation, sitz bath
- **Rose** is excellent for all female problems in preference to all other oils. Although expensive it is well worth the investment. It is cleansing, purifying, regulating and tonic
- Frigidity
- Heavy periods
- Impotence – increases the sperm count
- Irregular menstruation
- Sterility
- Vaginal discharges
- Women with a tendency to miscarriage

Neurological/emotional
Use in bath, compress, diffuser, inhalation, massage
- Depression – especially post-natal
- Frigidity and impotence
- Insomnia
- Nervous system
- Sadness
- Shock and grief

Skin care
Use in bath, compress, massage
- *All* skin care
- Dry skin
- Mature skin
- Redness or inflammation
- Sensitive skin
- Thread veins
- Wrinkles

Blends well with bergamot, geranium, neroli

Rosemary

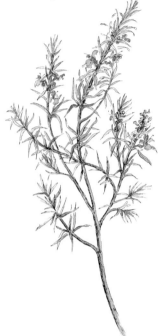

Latin name	Rosmarinus officinalis
Family	Labiatae
Note	Middle
Essence from	Leaves and flowering tops
Fragrance	Clean, eucalyptus-like, fiery, invigorating

Principal properties and indications

Keywords

- Diuretic
- Healing
- Pain-relieving
- Restorative
- Stimulating
- an important oil with a multitude of uses

Circulatory
Use in bath, diffuser, inhalation, massage

- Anaemia
- Arteriosclerosis
- Helps to normalise a high cholesterol level
- Lymphatic congestion
- Palpitations
- Regulates blood pressure
- Heart tonic — mildly stimulating

Digestive
Use in bath, compress, diffuser, inhalation, massage

- Colitis
- Diarrhoea
- Flatulence
- Hangover
- Indigestion
- Liver/gall bladder conditions
- Stomach pains

Genito-urinary
Use in bath, compress, massage, sitz bath

- Fluid retention
- Painful periods
- Vaginal discharge

Head
Use in bath, compress, diffuser, inhalation, massage

- Dandruff and hair loss
- Fainting
- Headache and migraine
- Loss of smell
- Oily hair

Muscular/joints
Use in bath, compress, massage

- Arthritis
- Gout
- Muscular aches and pains
- Rheumatism
- Stiff, overworked muscles

Neurological/emotional
Use in bath, diffuser, inhalation, massage

- All conditions where there is a reduction or loss of function – e.g. loss of memory, stroke
- Clears the mind
- Hysteria
- Lack of energy and lethargy
- Sadness
- Tonic
- Uplifting

Respiratory
Use in bath, compress, diffuser, inhalation, massage

- Asthma
- Bronchitis
- Catarrh
- Colds
- Flu
- Whooping cough

Skin care
Use in bath, compress, massage

- Abscess
- Acne
- Dermatitis
- Dry and ageing skin
- Eczema
- Rejuvenating
- Scabies and lice
- Wounds and burns
- Wrinkles

Contraindications
Do not use *excessively* in cases of epilepsy

Blends well with citrus oils (especially bergamot), frankincense, lavender, peppermint

Sandalwood (Mysore)

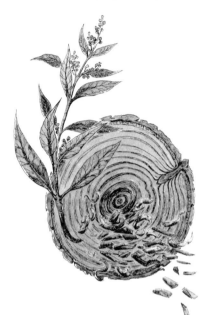

Latin name	Santalum album
Family	Santalaceae
Note	Base
Essence from	Wood of tree
Fragrance	Heady, heavy, oriental, sweet, warm, woody

Principal properties and indications
Keywords

- Antiseptic
- Aphrodisiac
- Fluid reducing
- Healing
- Soothing
- Uplifting

Genito-urinary
Use in bath, massage, sitz bath

- **Sandalwood** is one of the best oils to use for genito-urinary infections
- Cystitis
- Fluid retention

- Vaginal discharges of all kinds

Neurological/emotional
Use in bath, diffuser, inhalation, massage

- Anxiety
- Depression
- Frigidity and impotence
- Insomnia
- Nervous tension

Respiratory
Use in bath, diffuser, inhalation, massage

- Bronchitis
- Catarrh
- Coughs (especially dry)
- Laryngitis and other throat disorders (gargle with two drops in a glass of water)
- Respiratory tract infections

Skin care
Use in bath, compress massage

- *All* skin care
- Acne and oily skin
- Broken veins
- Cracked and chapped skin
- Dry, dehydrated skin

Blends well with almost all oils especially bergamot, cypress, neroli, rose

Tangerine

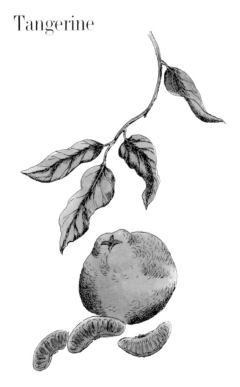

Latin name	Citrus reticulata
Family	Rutaceae
Note	Top
Essence from	Rind of the fruit
Fragrance	Bergamot-like, exotic, refreshing, sweet, tangy

Principal properties and indications
Keywords

- Calming
- Refreshing
- Revitalising
- Uplifting
- Tonic
- **Tangerine** is low in toxicity and is very therapeutic for young children and pregnant women. Everyone adores the fragrance of **tangerine**

Digestive
Use in bath, compress, massage
- Flatulence
- Hiccoughs
- Indigestion
- Liver problems
- Obesity and lymphatic blockage
- Stomach pains

Neurological/emotional
Use in bath, diffuser, inhalation, massage
- Anxiety
- Depression
- Hysteria
- Insomnia
- Nervous tension
- Shock and grief

Blends well with lavender, neroli

Tea-tree

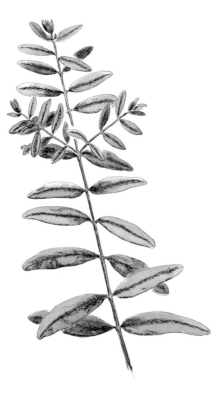

Latin name	*Melaleuca alterniflora*
Family	Myrtaceae
Note	Top
Essence from	Leaves
Fragrance	Antiseptic, camphor-like, sharp, strong

Principal properties and indications
Keywords
- Antiseptic
- Anti-fungal
- Anti-infectious
- Stimulating. Its vast range of uses and low toxicity makes it a must for a first aid kit

Circulatory
Use in bath, diffuser, inhalation, massage
- Aids
- Glandular fever
- ME (myalgic encephalomyelitis)
- **Tea-tree** boosts the immune system possibly more effectively than any other oil

Digestive
Use in bath, compress, massage
- Candida
- Indigestion
- Infections of the digestive tract
- Intestinal parasites

Genito-urinary
Use in bath, massage, sitz bath
- Cystitis
- Itching
- Thrush
- Vaginal discharge and infection

Thyme

Head
Use as a gargle (2 drops in a glass of water) and as a final hair rinse (2 drops)

- Cold sores (apply neat)
- Dandruff
- Gum infections
- Mouth ulcers
- Throat infections

Respiratory
Use in bath, compress, diffuser, inhalation, massage

- Bronchitis
- Catarrh
- Colds
- Flu
- Sinusitis

Skin care
Use in bath, compress, massage

- Abscess
- Acne
- Chickenpox
- All cuts and wounds
- Foot problems – athlete's foot, corns, cracked skin, smelly feet
- Herpes (anal, genital and oral)
- Infected wounds and ulcers
- Psoriasis
- Rashes
- Shingles, blisters

Blends well with bergamot, lavender, myrrh

Latin name	Thymus vulgaris
Family	Labiatae
Note	Middle
Essence from	Leaves and flowering tops
Fragrance	Hot, penetrating, powerful, sharp

Principal properties and indications
Keywords
- Antiseptic
- Strong
- Stimulant

Circulatory
Use in bath, massage

- Anaemia
- Depleted immune system – works excellently with **tea-tree**
- low blood pressure
- poor circulation

Digestive
Use in bath, diffuser, inhalation, massage

- Anorexia
- Flatulence
- Loss of appetite
- Poor digestion
- Worms

Genito-urinary
Use in bath, massage, sitz bath

- Absence of menstruation
- Fluid retention
- Urinary tract infections
- Vaginal discharges

Head
Use as a gargle (2 drops in a glass of water)

- Gum infections
- Mouth infections
- Sore throat

Muscular/joints
Use in bath, compress, massage

- Arthritis
- Gout
- Rheumatism

Neurological/emotional
Use in bath, diffuser, inhalation, massage

- Anxiety
- Depression
- Insomnia
- Memory improvement
- Nervous exhaustion
- Physical and mental debility (good for convalescence)

Respiratory
Use in bath, diffuser, inhalation, massage

- Asthma
- Bronchitis
- Cough
- Sinusitis
- Throat infections
- Whooping cough

Skin care
Use in bath, compress, massage

- Boils and carbuncles
- Scabies and lice
- Sores and wounds

Contraindications

1 Avoid during pregnancy

2 Take care with sensitive skins

Blends well with bergamot and other citrus oils, rosemary, tea-tree

Ylang ylang

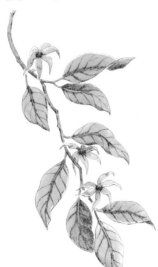

Latin name	*Canaga odorata*
Family	*Anonaceae*
Note	Base
Essence from	Flowers
Fragrance	Exotic, luxurious, sweet

Principal properties and indications

Keywords
- Antidepressant
- Aphrodisiac
- Euphoric
- Soothing
- Sometimes referred to as 'poor man's **jasmine'**

Circulatory
Use in bath, compress, diffuser, inhalation, massage
- Abnormally fast breathing
- Irregular heart beat
- Palpitations
- Reduces high blood pressure (Hypertension)

Neurological/emotional
Use in bath, diffuser, inhalation, massage
- Anxiety and tension
- Depression
- Fear
- Impotence and frigidity
- Insomnia
- Shock
- States of anger

Skin care
Use in bath, compress, massage
- All skin care
- Oily skin

Blends well with all citrus oils

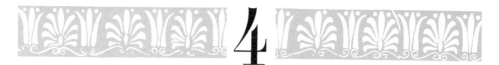

4

AROMATHERAPY FOR COMMON AILMENTS. A THERAPEUTIC INDEX

Circulatory disorders

Aids
Chamomile, lavender, tea-tree

Anaemia
Black pepper, chamomile, lemon, peppermint, rosemary, thyme

Arteriosclerosis
Black pepper, ginger, juniper, lemon, rosemary

Chilblains
Lemon

Fever
Black pepper, chamomile, eucalyptus, ginger, juniper, lavender, peppermint

Glandular fever
Cypress, lavender, lemon, tea-tree, thyme

Haemorrhoids
Cypress, geranium, juniper

Heart
- *False angina*   Neroli
- *Irregular heart beat (tachycardia)*   Ylang ylang
- *Tonic*   Lavender, marjoram, neroli, rose

High blood pressure
Chamomile, lavender, lemon, marjoram, neroli, ylang ylang

High cholesterol
Rosemary, thyme

Immune system booster
Chamomile, lavender, lemon, tea-tree, thyme

Low blood pressure
Rosemary, thyme

Lymphatic congestion
Chamomile, cypress, fennel, juniper, rosemary, tangerine

ME (myalgic encephalomyelitis)
Cypress, lavender, rosemary, tea-tree, thyme

Palpitations
Lavender, neroli, rose, rosemary, ylang ylang

Poor circulation
Benzoin, black pepper, cypress, ginger, lemon, tangerine, thyme

Varicose veins
Cypress, lemon

Digestive disorders

Anorexia nervosa
Bergamot, fennel, lavender, neroli, tangerine, thyme

Bulimia
Bergamot, geranium, jasmine, lavender, neroli, rose

Candida albicans infection
Tea-tree

Colic
Bergamot, black pepper, chamomile, clary sage, fennel, juniper, lavender, lemongrass, marjoram, peppermint

Colitis
Bergamot, black pepper, chamomile, lavender, lemongrass, neroli, rosemary

Constipation
Black pepper, fennel, marjoram, rose, rosemary

Diabetes
Eucalyptus, geranium, juniper

Diarrhoea
Black pepper, cajeput, chamomile, cypress, eucalyptus, geranium, ginger, lavender, lemon, myrrh, neroli (stress-induced), peppermint, rosemary, sandalwood

Fistula (anal)
Lavender

Flatulence
Bergamot, black pepper, chamomile, fennel, ginger, juniper, lavender,

lemon, lemongrass, marjoram, myrrh, neroli, peppermint, rosemary, tangerine, thyme

Food poisoning
Black pepper, fennel, juniper

Gall bladder
Bergamot, chamomile, geranium, lemon, peppermint, rose, rosemary

Hang-over
Fennel, juniper, rosemary

Heartburn
Black pepper, lemon (gastric antacid)

Hiccoughs
Basil, fennel, tangerine

Indigestion
Basil, bergamot, chamomile, cajeput, fennel, ginger, juniper, lavender, lemongrass, marjoram, myrrh, neroli (nervous), peppermint, rosemary, tangerine

Liver
Chamomile, cypress, geranium, lavender, lemon, peppermint, rose, rosemary, tangerine

Loss of appetite
Bergamot, black pepper, chamomile, fennel, ginger, juniper, peppermint, thyme

Nausea and vomiting
Basil, black pepper, chamomile, fennel, ginger, lavender, peppermint

Obesity
Fennel, juniper, lemon, rosemary

Sluggish digestion
Black pepper, fennel, juniper, peppermint

Spleen
Black pepper, chamomile, rosemary, thyme

Stomach pains
Chamomile, fennel, ginger, lavender, marjoram, peppermint, rosemary

Stomach ulcers
Chamomile, lemon

Travel sickness
Ginger, peppermint

Worms and intestinal parasites
Bergamot, chamomile, eucalyptus, geranium, juniper, lavender, myrrh, rosemary, tea-tree, thyme

Genito-urinary disorders

Childbirth
Clary sage, jasmine, lavender, neroli

Cystitis
Bergamot, cajeput, eucalyptus, juniper, lavender, sandalwood, tea-tree

Difficulty in passing urine
Juniper

Discharges
Bergamot, frankincense, lavender, marjoram, myrrh, rose, rosemary, sandalwood, tea-tree, thyme

Enuresis (bed-wetting)
Cypress

Excessive sexual impulses
Marjoram

Fluid retention
Chamomile, cypress, eucalyptus, fennel, geranium, juniper, lavender, lemon, lemongrass, rosemary, sandalwood, thyme

Frigidity and impotence
Clary sage, jasmine, neroli, rose, ylang ylang

Insufficiency of milk in nursing mothers
Fennel, jasmine, lemongrass

Itching (vaginal)
Bergamot, chamomile, tea-tree

Kidney infections and stones
Chamomile, eucalyptus, fennel, geranium, juniper, lemon, sandalwood

Menopause
Chamomile, cypress, fennel, geranium, jasmine, lavender, rose

Menstruation
- *Heavy blood loss*   Chamomile, cypress, geranium, rose
- *Irregular*   Chamomile, marjoram, rose
- *Painful*   Chamomile, cajeput, clary sage, cypress, jasmine, juniper, lavender, marjoram, peppermint, rose, rosemary
- *Scanty*   Chamomile, clary sage, fennel, juniper, lavender, myrrh, peppermint, rose, thyme

Oestrogen (stimulates body to produce)
Fennel

PMT
Chamomile, cypress, geranium, lavender, marjoram, rose

Prostate enlargement
Jasmine, juniper

Sterility
Geranium, rose

Thrush
Bergamot, frankincense, lavender, lemon, myrrh, tea-tree

Tonic for the womb
Clary sage, jasmine, rose

Urinary infections
Bergamot, cajeput, eucalyptus, juniper, sandalwood, thyme

Head disorders

Catarrh
Basil, eucalyptus, black pepper, frankincense, lavender, myrrh, tea-tree

Cold sores
Lavender, tea-tree

Earache
Basil, chamomile, lavender

Fainting and vertigo
Basil, black pepper, lavender, peppermint, rosemary

Gum infections (e.g. gingivitis)
Chamomile, lemon, myrrh, tea-tree, thyme

Hair and scalp
• *Dandruff*   Chamomile, juniper, lavender, lemon, patchouli, tea-tree, thyme
• *Dry*   Geranium, lavender, rosemary, sandalwood
• *Lice*   Lavender, rosemary, tea-tree
• *Loss of hair*   Lavender, rosemary
• *Oily*   Bergamot, clary sage, cypress, geranium, lemon, lemongrass, juniper, rosemary, thyme
• *Sensitive scalp*   Chamomile, lavender

Headache and migraine
Basil, chamomile, lavender, marjoram, peppermint, rosemary

Loss of smell
Rosemary

Mouth and tongue inflammation
Lemon, myrrh

Mouth infections and ulcers
Lemon, myrrh, tea-tree, thyme

Nasal polyps
Basil

Neuralgia
Basil, black pepper, chamomile, eucalyptus, geranium, peppermint

Rhinitis and sinusitis
Basil, cajeput, eucalyptus, lavender, peppermint, tea-tree, thyme

Teething pains and toothache
Chamomile, peppermint

Muscular and joint disorders

Aches and pains
Black pepper, chamomile, eucalyptus, frankincense, ginger, juniper, lavender, lemon, marjoram, peppermint, rosemary, thyme

Arthritis
Benzoin, black pepper, chamomile, eucalyptus, ginger, juniper, lavender, lemon, marjoram, peppermint, rosemary, thyme

Bruises
Chamomile, geranium, lavender, marjoram

Fibrositis
Black pepper, eucalyptus, lavender, peppermint, rosemary

Gout
Juniper, lemon, rosemary, thyme

Inflammation
Chamomile, lavender

Lack of muscle tone
Lavender, lemongrass, rosemary

Rheumatism
Black pepper, chamomile, eucalyptus, ginger, juniper, lavender, lemon, marjoram, peppermint, rosemary, thyme

Sprains and strains
Black pepper, chamomile, eucalyptus, ginger, lavender, marjoram, peppermint, rosemary

Stiffness
Black pepper, chamomile, eucalyptus, lavender, marjoram, rosemary

Neurological and emotional disorders

Alcoholism
Fennel

Anger
Chamomile, ylang ylang

Anorexia nervosa
Basil, benzoin, bergamot, geranium, jasmine, juniper, lavender, marjoram, neroli, patchouli, sandalwood, tangerine, thyme, ylang ylang

Apathy and lethargy
Jasmine, patchouli, rosemary

Change
Cypress (enables you to accept it), frankincense (enables you to move on)

Coldness
Benzoin, black pepper, frankincense, rose

Comfort
Benzoin, black pepper, cypress, rose

Confidence (lack of)
Ginger, jasmine

Courage
Black papper, fennel, ginger

Depression
Basil, bergamot, chamomile, clary sage, geranium, jasmine, lavender, neroli, patchouli, rose, sandalwood, tangerine, thyme, ylang ylang

Exhaustion
Benzoin (mental, emotional, physical) clary sage (nervous, physical, sexual), eucalyptus, juniper (emotional and nervous depletion), lavender, thyme

Fearful
Jasmine, neroli, frankincense, sandalwood, ylang ylang

Frigidity and impotence
Clary sage, jasmine, neroli, patchouli, peppermint, rose, sandalwood, ylang ylang

Grief
Benzoin, cypress, frankincense, marjoram, neroli, rose, tangerine

Hysteria and panic
Chamomile, clary sage, lavender, neroli, marjoram

Inability to concentrate
Basil, peppermint, rosemary

Indecision
Basil, patchouli

Insomnia
Chamomile, lavender, marjoram, neroli, rose, sandalwood, tangerine, ylang ylang

Irritability
Chamomile, cypress, lavender, thyme

Jealousy
Rose

Loneliness
Benzoin

Memory (poor)
Basil, ginger, juniper, rosemary, thyme

Mental fatigue (clears the mind)
Basil, peppermint, rosemary

Mood swings
Chamomile, geranium, lavender

Negativity
Jasmine, juniper

Nervous tension
Basil, cypress, marjoram, neroli, patchouli, rose, sandalwood, tangerine

Neuralgia
Basil, black pepper, chamomile, eucalyptus, geranium, peppermint

Obsessions
Frankincense

Oversensitivity
Basil, black pepper, chamomile, cypress, geranium, lavender

Sadness
Benzoin, jasmine, rose

Sedative
Bergamot, chamomile, clary sage, frankincense

Self-obsession
Rose

Shock
Neroli, peppermint, rose, tangerine, ylang ylang

Uplifting
Bergamot, clary sage, jasmine

Respiratory disorders

Asthma
Benzoin, cajeput, cypress, eucalyptus, frankincense, lavender, lemon, myrrh, peppermint, rosemary, thyme

Breath (fast)
Frankincense, lavender

Breath (shortness of)
Fennel, frankincense, lavender

Bronchitis
Benzoin, cajeput, eucalyptus, fennel, frankincense, lavender, lemon, myrrh, peppermint, rosemary, sandalwood, tea-tree, thyme

Catarrh
Benzoin, black pepper, eucalyptus, frankincense, ginger, lavender, lemon, myrrh, rosemary, sandalwood, tea-tree

Coughs and colds
Benzoin, black pepper, cajeput, eucalyptus, frankincense, ginger, lavender, lemon, myrrh, peppermint, rosemary, sandalwood, tea-tree, thyme

Cough (whooping)
Cypress, lavender, rosemary, thyme

Emphysema
Eucalyptus, frankincense

Flu
Benzoin, black pepper, eucalyptus, fennel, frankincense, ginger, lavender, lemon, peppermint, rosemary, tea-tree

Hoarseness and loss of voice
Myrrh, sandalwood

Laryngitis
Benzoin, cajeput, eucalyptus, lemon, sandalwood

Phlegm
Benzoin, black pepper, eucalyptus

Sinusitis
Cajeput, eucalyptus, lavender, lemon, tea-tree, thyme

Tonsillitis and throat infections
Benzoin, cajeput, eucalyptus, geranium, ginger, lavender, lemon, sandalwood

Skin disorders

Acne
Bergamot, chamomile, juniper, lavender, lemongrass, patchouli, peppermint, rosemary, sandalwood, tea-tree

Ageing skin
Clary sage, frankincense, lavender, myrrh, neroli, patchouli, rose, rosemary

Allergy
Chamomile, lavender, patchouli

Athlete's Foot
Lavender, myrrh, patchouli, tea-tree

Bleeding
Geranium

Boils and carbuncles
Bergamot, chamomile, lavender, lemon, rosemary, tea-tree, thyme

Broken capillaries
Cypress, neroli, rose, sandalwood

Bruises
Chamomile, geranium, lavender, marjoram

Burns
Chamomile, eucalyptus, lavender, geranium

Cellulite
Cypress, fennel, juniper, lemon

Chapped and cracked skin
Benzoin, myrrh, patchouli, sandalwood, tea-tree

Combination skin
Geranium, lavender, neroli

Cuts
Eucalyptus, lavender, lemon, tea-tree

Dermatitis
Benzoin, juniper, lavender, patchouli, peppermint, rosemary

Dry skin
Chamomile, clary sage, geranium, jasmine, lavender, neroli, rose, rosemary, sandalwood

Eczema
Bergamot, chamomile, geranium, juniper, lavender, myrrh, patchouli, rosemary

Herpes
Bergamot, eucalyptus, lemon, tea-tree

Inflamed, red, irritated skin
Benzoin, chamomile, clary sage, geranium, lavender, myrrh, neroli, peppermint, rose

Mature skin
Clary sage, frankincense, lavender, myrrh, neroli, patchouli, rose, sandalwood

Measles
Eucalyptus

Oily and open pores
Bergamot, clary sage, cypress, geranium, juniper, lavender, lemon, lemongrass, sandalwood, tea-tree, ylang ylang

Perspiration
Cypress, lemongrass, tea-tree

Psoriasis
Bergamot, lavender, tea-tree

Rejuvenative
Frankincense, lavender, myrrh, neroli

Scabies
Lemon, lemongrass, peppermint, rosemary, thyme

Sensitive
Chamomile, geranium, jasmine, neroli, lavender, rose

Sunburn
Clary sage, lavender, peppermint

Ulcers
Frankincense, geranium, juniper, lavender, myrrh, tea-tree

Varicose veins
Cypress, lemon

Warts and verrucae
Lemon, tea-tree

Wounds and sores
Benzoin, frankincense, geranium, juniper, myrrh, patchouli, tea-tree, thyme

Wrinkles
Clary sage, frankincense, myrrh, patchouli, rose, rosemary

5

AURAS AND CHAKRAS

What is the aura?

The human aura is like a protective electro-magnetic energy field completely surrounding our physical body. It is made up of many different colours and composed of several layers. The size and shape of the aura will vary enormously from one individual to another. Some psychics claim to be able to see it – I believe that everyone can at least feel it and I have never had a student at the college on an aromatherapy course who was not able to sense it. If you are sceptical (and many are) then close your eyes and hold your hands a few inches away from another person's body. What you can feel emanating from the body is the aura (feel all around the body from the head to the toes). Notice any tingling sensations, feelings of warmth or coldness, any areas which feel stronger or weaker, congested or depleted. Incredible isn't it?

What is the purpose of the aura?

An aura is basically a protective skin acting like a two-way filter, providing protection from negative influences whilst allowing any positive influences to enter. Auras are healthier and more regular in shape in a balanced person than in an unbalanced one. If an unhealthy aura is present then the negative influences which enter will result in mental and physical tensions giving rise to all manner of diseases. The healthier a person is, the more regular his or her energy field will be.

A disturbed or unhealthy aura will:

- Shrink
- Become lop-sided
- Bulge out in some areas
- Feel rough and congested
- Darken or cloud over
- Develop holes through which energy leaks

What depletes the aura?

- Physical disease
- Emotional trauma
- Negative thoughts
- Drugs
- Alcohol
- Smoking
- Accidents ⎫
- Surgery ⎬ the memory remains in the aura
- Past illness ⎭

Where someone has a hole in their aura they will feel very depleted and lacking in energy since their energy is being lost through the hole. Sometimes you will meet people (or perhaps you have friends like it!) who leave you feeling drained, depleted, thoroughly depressed and perhaps even physically ill. Such people are 'energy vampires' who, often unintentionally, suck up and drain your energy.

If this occurs in everyday life, then it is not difficult to believe that it is likely to happen far more during an aromatherapy treatment when you are actually, probably unknowingly, working in the aura!

Massaging the aura with essential oils provides enormous benefits. It can help to eliminate bad memories, clear away past traumas and can even prevent disease from manifesting itself in the physical body.

If auras interest you then refer to the section on further reading. If you find the concept of auras difficult to accept, then perhaps you should look at some Kirlian work where auras are actually photographed.

In Kirlian photography, electrical interference patterns are recorded using high voltage, high frequency means. The image produced can be used as a counselling tool to monitor what is happening in the subtle energy field which surrounds the human body and to show some of the emotional and physical changes that can occur when people are under stress.

According to the system of Philippe Pien of the Centre Européen d'Etudes Biologiques, the hands represent the person's spiritual and emotional side and are a valuable source of analysis for the counsellor.

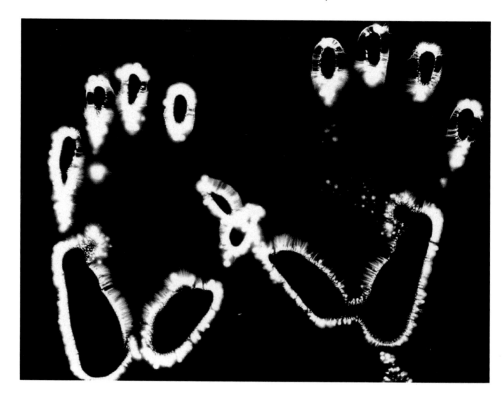

The flares on the fingers represent the person's spirituality, creativity, well-being etc. If they appear blocked, as in the photograph on page 64, it could suggest that the person is unable to express this side of the personality to its full potential and is feeling suffocated by his or her environment. Once such an analysis has been made, suitable therapies, such as aromatherapy, or even something as simple as gentle exercise or talking about problems, can be suggested.

The feet represent the person's physical side and by looking at the way the toes appear, the counsellor can assess how different parts of the body are working. Each toe represents a different part of the body and by analysing areas which do not appear clearly on the Kirlian photograph the counsellor can suggest possible problem areas and recommend suitable therapies or treatments.

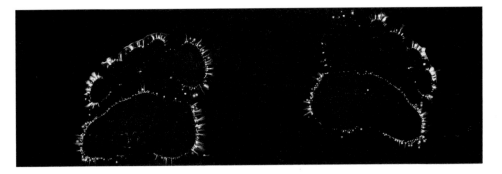

Protecting yourself

If you are intuitive, and most individuals (both male and female) are, it is important that you know how to protect yourself prior to the aromatherapy treatment to avoid feeling weak and depleted. Even if you are not aware of your intuition I think that you will find that your intuition will grow. I know that mine certainly has! When I first heard of auras and chakras I thought that I was talking to a 'nutcase'! But over the years I have been fortunate in that my intuition has developed enormously.

Ground yourself prior to a treatment by ensuring that both feet are firmly placed on the ground. You can imagine that there are roots on the the soles of your feet growing deep down into the earth.

Imagine that white healing light (or any colour you wish) is pouring down from the sky and surrounding your whole body. Feel that you are protected within this light as you work.

At the end of the treatment you should always ensure that you are grounded and then hold your hands under *cold* running water or even dip the arms up to the elbow in water. Cold water is cleansing both physically and psychically.

You will undoubtedly find your own favourite methods of protecting yourself when the need arises – some people imagine golden cloaks around them.

What are the chakras?

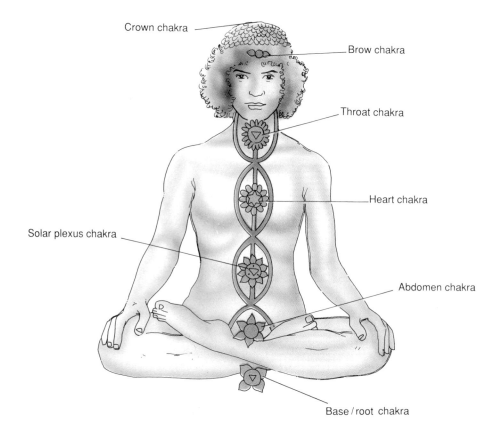

Crown chakra

Brow chakra

Throat chakra

Heart chakra

Solar plexus chakra

Abdomen chakra

Base / root chakra

The 'chakras' are like constantly revolving wheels of energy which penetrate both the aura and the physical body. They rotate in a clockwise direction and also open and close. There are hundreds of chakras throughout the body (opinions vary as to the number which exist and terminology) but most agree that there are *seven* major chakras.

I will describe the chakras in brief, stating the position, colour, the endocrine gland which that chakra is thought to influence (opinions vary on this too) and physiological and psychological disorders which may result if that particular chakra is out of balance.

Base/root chakra (base of the spine)

- *Colour*   Red – symbolically has four petals
- *Connections with*   Gonads (ovaries, testes)
- *Physical imbalances include*   Bladder problems, cancer, colon problems (e.g. constipation), female/male reproductive organ problems, sciatica problems
- *Psychological imbalances include*   Dependent personality, identity crisis, inability to ground oneself, inability to release negativity, sexual perversion, promiscuity, lack of self-esteem, sense of inferiority, shame, guilt, regret

This is the centre of surviving, grounding and letting go. It may be disturbed temporarily during stages of sexual transition such as puberty, pregnancy, menopause, or after gynaecological operations such as hysterectomy.

Abdomen chakra (abdominal area)

- *Colour*   Orange – symbolically has six petals
- *Connections with*   Pancreas/spleen
- *Physical imbalances*   Anaemia, allergies, diabetes, digestive problems, kidney problems, pancreas/spleen problems, poor digestion, poor food combination, ulcers
- *Psychological imbalances*   Depression, hysteria, lack of motivation, lack of energy, greed, envy, jealousy, resentment

Solar plexus chakra (apex of rib cage – energy balancer)

- *Colour*   Yellow – symbolically has 10 petals
- *Connected with*   Adrenal glands
- *Physical imbalances*   Adrenal problems, anorexia, arthritis, bulimia, liver problems, obesity
- *Psychological imbalances*   Addictive personality, egocentricity, excess of emotions, fear, frustration, inability to relax, insecurity, manic-depressive behaviour, phobias, poor concentration, schizophrenia, sleep problems, self-centred, tension, uneasiness

Heart chakra (centre of chest – unconditional love)

- *Colour*   Green – symbolically has 12 petals
- *Connected with*   Thymus gland
- *Physical imbalances include*   Asthma, blood pressure problems, circulatory problems, heart problems, hyperventilation, lung and respiratory disorders, immune system problems, strokes
- *Psychological imbalances include*   Unable to love oneself and therefore unable to love others, self-destructive tendencies, 'hurt' feelings, insecure, competitive, lack of compassion and understanding, extreme emotional sensitivity

Throat chakra (centre of throat – communication)

- *Colour*   Blue – symbolically has 16 petals
- *Connected with*   Thyroid gland
- *Physical imbalances include*   Thyroid/parathyroid problems, throat problems, neck and shoulder problems, non-stop verbal chatter
- *Psychological imbalances include*   Inability to express oneself, stuttering, negative attitude towards others causing an inability to integrate with them, self-destructive tendencies

Brow chakra (centre of forehead – third eye)

- *Colour*   Indigo – symbolically has 96 petals
- *Connected with*   Pituitary gland
- *Physical imbalances include*   Headaches, sinus problems, eye or visual disorders, brain tumours, pituitary problems, memory disorders, dizziness
- *Psychological imbalances include*   Depression, extreme confusion, hallucinations, identity crisis, inability to focus, living in a fantasy world, lack of vision, lack of intuition, mental imbalance, mood swings, self-absorption

Crown chakra (crown of head)

- *Colour*   Violet – symbolically has 972 petals
- *Connected with*   Pineal gland
- *Physical imbalances include*   Migraine headache, epilepsy, Parkinson's disease, brain tumours, neuritis
- *Psychological imbalances include*   Gullible, nightmares, closed mind, fear of opening up to spiritual levels, fear of insanity and losing control

The relevance of the chakras to aromatherapy lies in the ability of pure essential oils to profoundly influence, unblock and balance the chakras. Each individual will have his or her own ideas as to which oils have an affinity for which chakras and there are really no rules. I have listed some suggestions but you can make up your own mind.

Base chakra
Oils to ground, often base notes: Benzoin, frankincense, myrrh, patchouli, vertivert. Aphrodisiac oils: Jasmine, neroli, rose, sandalwood, ylang ylang. Anaphrodisiac oils: marjoram.

Abdomen chakra
Oils to improve digestion and energy: Bergamot, black pepper, fennel, ginger, marjoram, peppermint, rosemary, thyme

Solar plexus chakra
Oils to relax, cleanse, balance mood swings and encourage sleep: Bergamot, Roman chamomile, cypress, geranium, juniper (cleanses), lavender, lemon, neroli, sage (protects)

Heart chakra
Oils to open up the heart to allow the establishment of bonds with others: Benzoin, bergamot, black pepper, cypress, frankincense, melissa, neroli, rose (especially Bulgarian rose otto), vertivert, ylang ylang

Throat chakra
Oils to encourage communication and confidence to express oneself: Benzoin, blue chamomile, black pepper, ginger, jasmine, myrrh, sandalwood

Brow chakra
Oils to encourage vision and clarify the mind: Basil, black pepper, clary sage, fennel, ginger, juniper, lavender, peppermint, rosemary, thyme

Crown chakra
Oils to dispel any fears to open up the mind to spiritual levels: Benzoin, frankincense, lavender, neroli, jasmine, rose, rosewood, sandalwood, ylang ylang

6

STEP-BY-STEP GUIDE TO GIVING AN AROMATHERAPY MASSAGE

An aromatherapy massage is undoubtedly the most effective way of deriving maximum benefit from essential oils. During the treatment, the healing energy of the hands and the oils join forces to melt away stresses and tensions and to affect profoundly the physical, emotional and spiritual levels.

The physical, emotional and spiritual history of an individual may be revealed before your eyes if you choose to look. Every body tells a story by reflecting memories of the past. Bodies do not usually move freely and without restriction but instead, often display signs of defensive 'armouring' and 'energy blockages'.

A child may experience a frightening fall. Although physically this could lead to only minor injuries, the 'fear' of the fall may mirror itself in the body. The shoulders would be held tightly in an elevated and forward position resulting in contraction of the chest muscles. Such 'body armouring' could eventually restrict the ability to breathe properly and such shallow breathing may create anxiety. After a car accident the bones may heal but the emotional trauma of the event may remain. The tissues and the nervous system appear to 'remember' both physical *and* emotional trauma.

Emotions may also accumulate even in the organs of the body. For instance, the liver may store anger and depression, the heart a fear of being hurt in love and the lungs may be a storage organ for unresolved grief.

During the aromatherapy massage, as your hands embark on their journey of discovery, alleviating knots and nodules and sore and sensitive areas, be prepared for the possibility of an emotional release. A painful memory may be given the opportunity to rise to the surface and release itself, enabling the energy to circulate freely through the body once more. Painful past incidents will not necessarily be recalled during the treatment but could be remembered within a few days, perhaps during a dream. Once the painful emotion is recalled, it is freed.

Setting the scene

Creating the right atmosphere

It is extremely important to pay particular attention to the environment in which the aromatherapy massage is to be performed if maximum benefit is to be derived from the treatment. Careful preparation and the right setting will make a good massage even better! The environment should be arranged so that both giver and receiver feel immediately relaxed, just by being there. Always ensure that all towels, cushions and oils are on hand so as not to lose contact and thus break the flow of the massage.

Pay careful attention to the following:

Solitude and peace
These are vital. Ensure that you choose a time when you will not be disturbed. Intrusions and distractions are extremely disconcerting, breaking your concentration and destroying the flow of your massage movements. Take the telephone off the hook and tell your friends and family not to enter the treatment room. You may decide to choose some soothing background music although this is a matter of personal preference. Some will prefer silence.

Cleanliness
This is essential too. Always wash your hands before the treatment as any stickiness will be instantly obvious to the receiver. Make sure that fingernails are short – trim them as far down as possible. Do not wear any jewellery on the hands.

Warmth
The room should be draught-free and very warm, yet well ventilated. Nothing will destroy a massage more quickly than physical coldness. It is impossible to relax when you feel cold. The room in which you give the massage should be heated prior to the treatment, and as the body temperature will drop, ensure that spare towels and blankets are at your disposal. All areas should be kept covered other than the part on which you are working. Warm your hands if they feel cold.

Lighting
Soft and subdued lighting will create the ideal atmosphere. Bright lights falling on the receiver's face will hardly induce relaxation and will cause tension around the eyes. Candlelight provides the perfect setting or you may wish to use a tinted bulb. Pale blue, green, peach, pink or lavender all have a beneficial effect.

Colour
The most therapeutic colours to have in the room are pastel shades – pale pink, blue, green, lavender or peach decor and towels are perfect for the occasion. These colours represent calmness, healing, love and nurturing. Colours such as red and black will tend to create unwanted emotions like anger, hate, restlessness, negativity and depression.

Clothes

Wear comfortable and loose-fitting clothes as you need to move around easily and the room in which you will be working will be very warm. White is the best colour to wear when giving a massage since it will reflect any negativity which is released from the individual being treated.

Wear flat shoes or, even better, go barefoot. The receiver should undress down to whatever level they feel comfortable with. Suggest they undress down to at least their underwear. Point out that any areas which are not being worked on will be covered up as this will create a sense of security and trust.

Finishing touches

Use some fresh flowers to add a pleasant aroma to the atmosphere or even diffuse an essential oil prior to the treatment. Crystals may also be employed to enhance the environment. These are healing in their own right, capable of drawing unbalanced energy out of the human body. In my treatment room I have a large piece of purple amethyst for absorbing any negativity which I cleanse at the end of each day with pure spring water.

Equipment

Massage surface

You may work on the floor using a firm yet well padded surface. This will allow you to give a massage wherever you desire. Place a large, thick piece of foam or two or three blankets or a thick duvet on the floor. Use plenty of cushions during the massage. When the receiver is lying on the back place one under the head and one under the knees to take the pressure off the lower back.

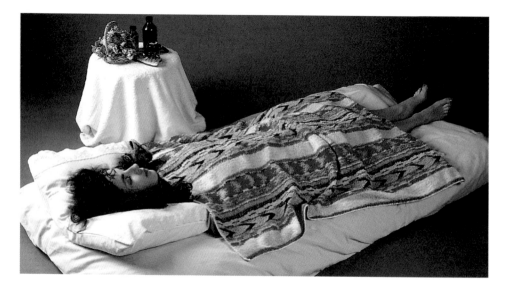

When the receiver is lying on the front place a cushion under the feet, one under the shoulders and perhaps one under the abdomen if desired.

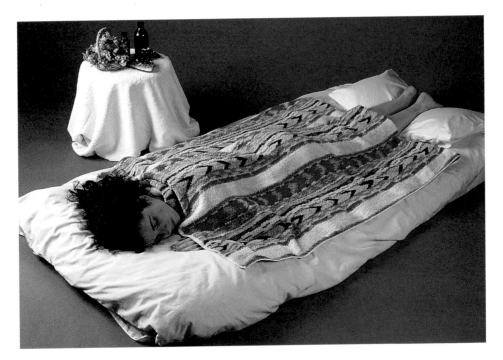

Ensure that you have something to kneel on to avoid sore knees. If you are unfortunate enough to be a back sufferer or have knee problems it may be a good idea to invest in a portable couch. It is far less tiring and makes the body readily accessible. You could try improvising by using the kitchen table if the height is comfortable for you. **Do not** use a bed as most are far too soft and are such an awkward height that you will need a massage yourself when you finish! Most mattresses are too soft for massage purposes as any pressure applied is absorbed by the mattress.

Oils

Blend the oil by referring to the chapter on aromatherapy treatment techniques and the therapeutic index. Ensure that you are using the appropriate dilution and that you are adopting my holistic approach by selecting at least one oil for any emotional imbalances. Allow the recipient to smell the blended oils bearing in mind that we are drawn to the essential oils which are beneficial to us at the time.

Always keep the oil within easy reach during the treatment. Do not use too much oil as you will be unable to make proper contact and the receiver will feel most uncomfortable and sticky. A complete treatment actually requires very little oil – just a few teaspoons. **Never** pour oil directly onto the body. Pour about half a teaspoon onto the palm of one hand and then rub your hands together to warm the oil slightly before applying it. When you require more lubricant keep one hand in contact with the body. Breaking contact destroys the continuity of the massage and creates a feeling of insecurity.

Your attitude and state of mind

Posture
Whether you are working on the floor or at a table, keep your back relaxed yet straight throughout the aromatherapy treatment. Remember that it should be as relaxing to give an aromatherapy massage as it is to receive one. With practice you will learn to avoid tensing the muscles so that the healing energy can flow freely through your hands and body.

Attunement
Your state of mind when giving an aromatherapy treatment is vital. The quality and success of a treatment depends upon having a calm state of mind. Do not attempt to give a massage when you are feeling angry, moody, anxious, depressed or unwell. Your negativity will be transmitted. Your complete attention must be devoted to the receiver. If you are worrying about your own problems and your mind is drifting then this will be communicated immediately.

Spend time consciously relaxing yourself prior to the treatment and, most importantly, be guided by your own intuition. Take a few deep breaths before the massage allowing all tension and anxiety to flow out of your body. Breathe in peace and breathe out love. Tune in to the person you are massaging. It will help to work with the eyes closed. Give yourself unselfishly to the massage. If necessary surround yourself before you begin with a white light for protection.

The treatment

This step-by-step guide will enable you to carry out an aromatherapy massage on your friends and family. I do urge you to work intuitively and to develop your own individual style. This aromatherapy routine is completely subjective – there is no 'correct' way to perform an aromatherapy massage. The treatment will concentrate on the important areas of the back, legs, feet, neck, shoulders, chest and face. For treatment of the abdomen and other areas please refer to my other book on *Massage* in this series. Obviously if you intend to use aromatherapy professionally then formal training with a reputable establishment is necessary (see Useful Addresses on page 112). This would entail the study of anatomy and physiology which is essential for professional use as well as specialised aromatherapy techniques and too complicated to be described here. Do not be tempted by a weekend course.

Back of body

Back and shoulders

The receiver should be lying on his or her front with pillows placed under the feet and shoulders, all other areas being completely covered with towels. The arms may be placed at the sides or may hang over the edge of the massage couch. The head may be turned to one side or, if this causes pain, then the forehead could be placed on the hands.

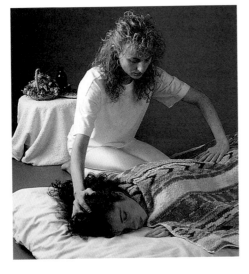

Step 1 – tuning in to the back
Before using any oil, position yourself at the side of the receiver (choose whichever side you feel most comfortable) placing one hand on top of the head and the other hand at the bottom of the spine. Gently rest them there for about a minute. This enables you to tune in and engenders a feeling of relaxation and trust in the receiver.

Step 2 – applying the oil
Draw back the towel slowly. Warm the oil slightly in the palms of your hands and working from the side of the body commence with both hands palms down at the bottom of the back, fingers pointing towards the head, one hand either side of the spine. Stroke firmly up towards the neck, over the shoulders and glide back to the starting point using no pressure on the return. Mould your hands to the contours of the body as you apply the oil.

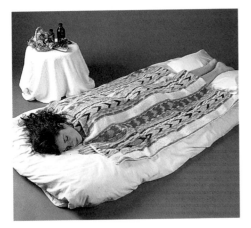

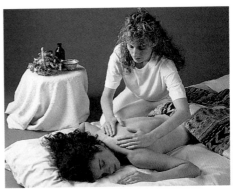

Step 3 – drawing energy down
Positioned at the side, bring the palms of the hands almost together to rest them with the little fingers on the centre of the spine imagining that your hands are a cup drawing healing white light down onto the receiver. Gradually unfold them so that one hand slides up the back towards the head and the other hand slides down to the base of the spine spreading out the energy as you stroke. The pressure is slow, yet firm and as the hands unfold, you may become aware of any areas of tension, changes in temperature, 'blockage' in energy and so forth. Breathe out as your hands slowly unfold leaning into the movement so that your whole body becomes involved. As the hands draw back to their starting point use no pressure at all.

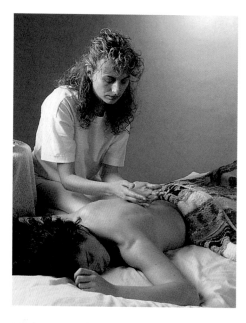

Place your hands in the same position but this time to the side of the spine to cover the side of the

back furthest away from you and then smooth out the side of the back nearest you.

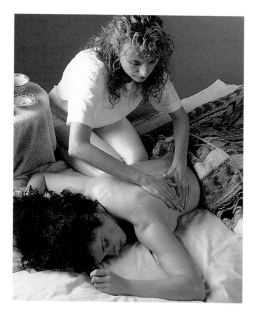

Repeat these three movements at least three times drawing the energy down and spreading it across the back.

These movements will calm and sedate (possibly sending the receiver to sleep!) engendering a sense of well-being and a relationship of trust and promoting the flow of energy.

Step 4 – awakening the spinal points
Place both thumbs on the same side of the spine as you are working, with the tips facing each other about one inch apart. Commence at the bottom of the back working close to the side of, but not directly onto, the spine itself. Press in gradually and deeply using your body weight to lean onto these points. Sustain the pressure for a few seconds then slowly release and proceed a little further up the back to the next set of points.

Always take care never to poke or prod these points sharply. Use these thumb pressures all the way up to the neck. Repeat at least twice. Without losing contact, position yourself on the other side of the receiver, to repeat these movements.

By pressing on these points you are exerting a positive influence on the vital organs and structures of the body, restoring and enhancing nerve supply, blood supply, lymphatic drainage and harmony.

In addition to dispersing energy this movement is also useful for breaking down knots and nodules, old scar tissue and fatty deposits.

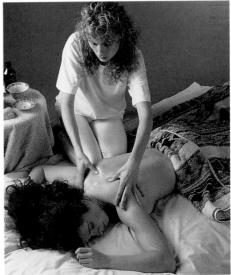

Step 6 – spinal thumb sliding

Place the balls of the thumbs in the dimples again and glide them up to the neck and back down again three times. This movement re-inforces the action of the last step.

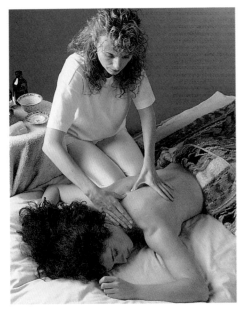

Step 5 – dispersing energy from the spinal points

Place the balls of the thumbs in the two dimples at the base of the spine and use small, slow, deep outward circular movements working up towards the base of the neck. Try to keep the thumbs parallel as you travel up the back dispersing the energy from the pressure points. Allow the hands to glide back to the starting point with no pressure. Repeat.

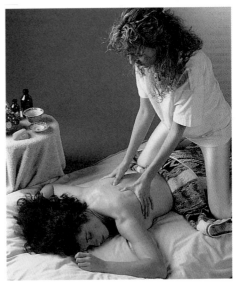

Step 7 – stretching the back

Place both forearms horizontally across the back. Gradually draw them apart so that one forearm is moving up towards the neck and the other forearm is moving down towards the buttocks. A wonderful movement for stretching the whole back.

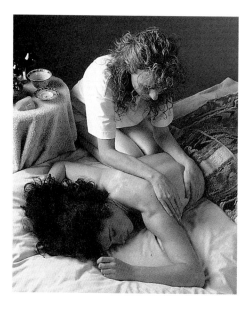

Step 8 – scooping up the muscle

Palms facing down, commence with both hands flat, on the same side of the lower back that you are working from. Scoop up and squeeze the muscle with both hands attempting to grasp as much flesh as possible. 'Scooping' is a

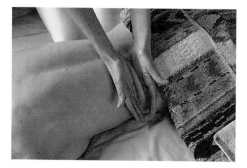

decongestive action designed to remove toxins from the deeper tissues. Fresh blood flows to the area bringing important nutrients to the muscles. Repeat on the other side.

Step 9 – hips and lower back and awakening the lower back

Place one hand flat on top of the other hand and using the whole of the hand make large figure of eight movements from the bottom of the spine circling over the right hip and then over the left hip. Repeat until the hips feel loosened.

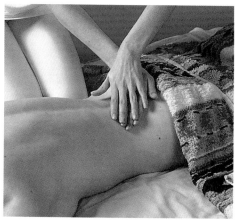

Step 10 – decongesting the lower back

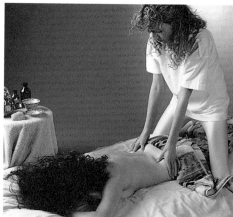

Locate the dimples and press and release around the sacrum (large triangular bone) and down and across the top of the pelvis three times. This may feel painful at first as the lumbar area is usually congested due to physical or emotional stress, bad posture or childbirth.

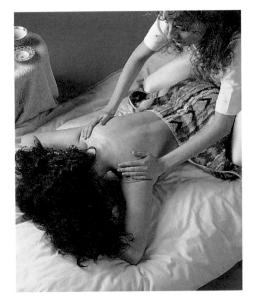

Step 11 – draining the lower back
Place both hands in the middle of the lower back, heels of the hands together with fingertips facing outwards. Stroke firmly out and over the hips. Glide the hands back using no pressure. Repeat several times.

Step 13 – decongesting the shoulders
Choose a shoulder blade and press and release with both thumbs working from the bottom of the shoulder blade up to the top and back again. (It is easier to commence at the bottom since the shoulder blade will usually stand out here.) Repeat on the other shoulder blade.

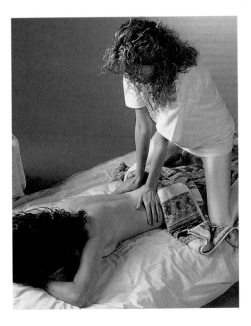

Step 12 – awakening the shoulders
Stroke up towards the shoulders bringing the towel with you so as to cover the lower back. Place your right hand flat down on the right shoulder blade and the left hand on the left shoulder blade. Make large outward circles with both hands simultaneously.

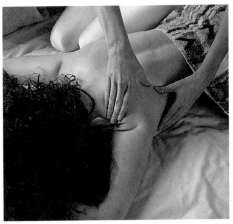

Step 14 – draining the shoulders
Positioned at the receiver's head, place both hands in the middle of

the upper back, heels of the hands together, fingertips facing outwards. Stroke firmly out and down towards the armpits. This will drain any toxins released into the axillary lymph nodes. Repeat several times.

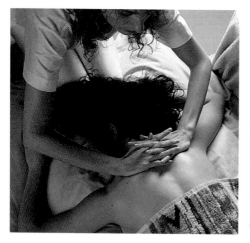

Step 15 – rocking the body

This is a marvellous movement for encouraging the release of tension and pent-up emotion. Those who find it easy to 'let go' will rock very easily. Start at the base of the spine placing one hand on each hip. Gently begin to rock the hips to and fro and once they are moving place your hands slightly higher up gradually rocking all the way up the body to the neck.

Step 16 – draining the toxins

This movement is performed down both sides of the body. Position both hands, fingertips pointing downwards, at the base of the spine on the side opposite to you. Push the toxins down towards the floor or couch and gently flick them away from the body. Work all the way up to the top of the shoulders. Do not lose contact as you move round to the other side of the receiver.

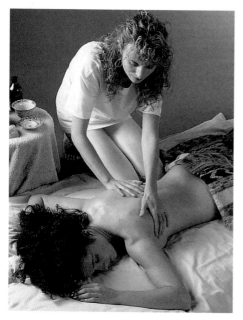

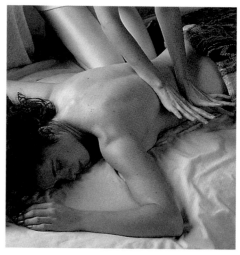

Step 17 – balancing the energies (chakras)

Take a deep breath, relax and close your eyes to increase your sensitivity. Place one hand on top of the head and place the other hand about two inches from the surface of the skin. Slowly scan the body from the head to the base of the spine. The hand which is acting as a detector should be totally relaxed to make it more effective. Simply sense and trust what comes through your hands. Be aware of changes in sensation, temperature, tingling, vibration, spinning and electric shock-type feelings.

In time you will be able to detect the chakras very easily. Try increasing the distance from the body to the scanning hand. If you feel that a chakra is out of balance then place one drop of an appropriate oil onto it (refer to Chapter 4). For instance if you pick up overactivity or congestion at the solar plexus chakra, reflecting an inability to relax and possible sleep problems, one drop of **Roman chamomile** could be used.

Rest one hand on the head and the other on the sacrum. Imagine that you are connecting the energies of the back. You may feel pulsation or a sudden rush of energy. If you feel absolutely nothing at first then do not despair. Often the receiver will experience more sensations than you do!

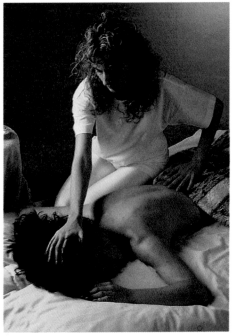

Completely cover the lower back with towels.

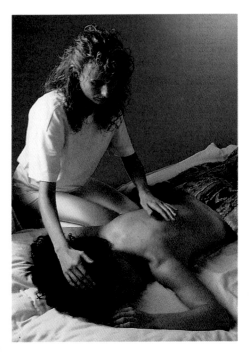

Back of the legs

Many aromatherapists use particular techniques for lymphatic drainage which are too complicated to describe in this book. However, as you massage be aware of any swelling at the ankles and at the back of the knees. Aromatherapy leg massage will improve circulation and lymphatic flow, relieve tired, aching legs and it can prevent varicose veins. **Cypress** and **lemon** are an excellent combination. Treatment is always performed up the legs towards the lymph glands in the groin area.

Step 1 – tuning in to the legs

Position yourself at the feet of the receiver. Rest cupped hands gently on each calf and take a few deep breaths holding them there for as long as you feel is necessary.

knee which can be a painful area particularly where there is lymphatic congestion. Take care over any varicose veins.

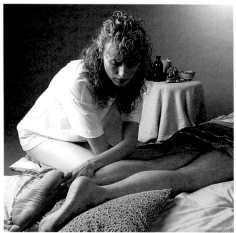

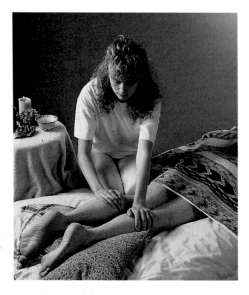

Step 3 – draining the lower leg

Lift up the foot supporting it in one hand and with the palm of the

Step 2 – awakening the legs with alternate hand stroking

Position yourself to the side of the receiver and draw back the towel to uncover the leg on which you are about to start working. Place cupped hands on the ankle nearest you. Using one hand stroke up from the ankle to the thigh. As it reaches the top of the thigh begin stroking upwards with the other hand. Repeat several times. Do not use pressure at the back of the

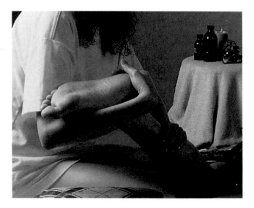

other hand stroke from the ankle firmly down towards the back of the bent knee. Repeat several times and then gently lower the leg.

Step 4 – liberating the lymph
Place both hands one on top of the other at the back of the knee. Using all of the fingers perform gentle circular movements to stimulate and activate the lymph glands at the back of the knee.

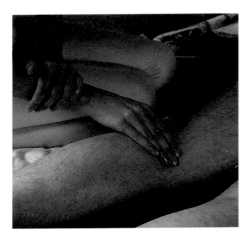

Step 5
Use the alternate hand stroking again to push any toxins which have been released towards the groin area.

Step 6 – unblocking the thigh

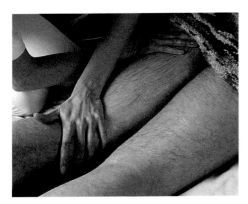

Commence with both hands cupped just above the back of the knee. Using alternate hands stroke firmly up to the thigh. You may also stroke both hands up together for added strength.

Step 7 – releasing the toxins
Many women have obstinate cellulite which is really toxic waste in the tissues. It is usually particularly bad on the outside of the thigh. Essential oils such as **cypress**, **fennel**, **juniper**, **lemon** and **rosemary** are particularly good for this condition and if you wish to reduce cellulite a combination of aromatherapy massage, skin brushing and a good diet is essential.

Pick up and squeeze the muscles of the inner thigh bringing it towards you first with one hand and then the other hand. Wring the middle muscle of the thigh from the same position. Fatty deposits will be broken down and waste products can be eliminated.

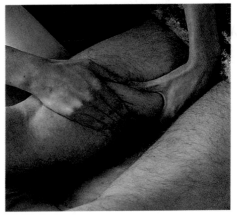

Step 8
Move round to the other side of the receiver and wring the other thigh. This area can be worked

upon very firmly to encourage release of toxins.

sacrum and the other gently on the ankle. Imagine that you are releasing any energy blockages and connecting the whole leg.

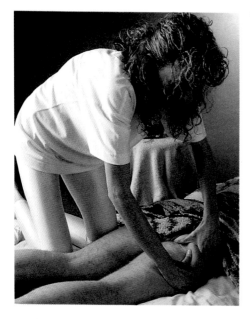

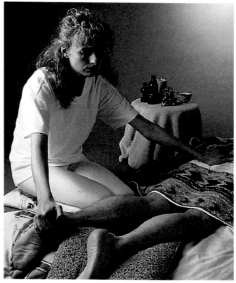

Step 9 – connecting the leg
Cover the leg with the towel and place one hand on the hip or

Repeat on the other leg.

Front of the body

Ask the receiver to turn over. Place one pillow under the head and one under the knees. Use more pillows if necessary.

Foot and lower leg

Step 1 – tuning in to the feet
Position yourself at the feet of the receiver and place one hand on the top of each foot. Breathe deeply holding gently onto the feet for about 30 seconds or as long as you feel is necessary.

Step 2 – awakening the foot
Stroke the entire foot firmly using both hands working from the toes

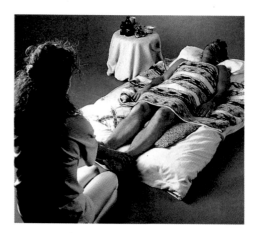

to the top of the foot. Slide around the ankle bones and glide back.

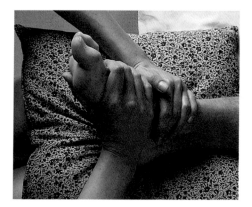

Step 3 – decongesting the foot
Supporting the foot with one hand use the knuckles of the other hand to make firm circular movements over the entire sole of the foot.

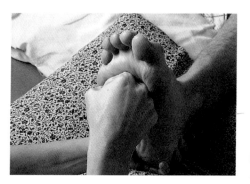

Step 4 – decongesting the ankle

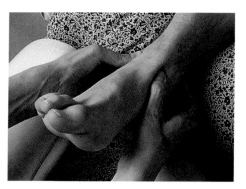

Stroke up to the ankle and make small, deep circular movements with the thumbs all around the ankle. This movement is excellent for reducing fluid.

Step 5 – awakening the front of the leg
Position yourself at the side of the receiver drawing back the towel to reveal the leg. Commence at the ankle with cupped hands and stroke the hands alternately up towards the thigh moulding to the contours of the leg. As one hand reaches the top of the thigh the other hand begins to stroke.

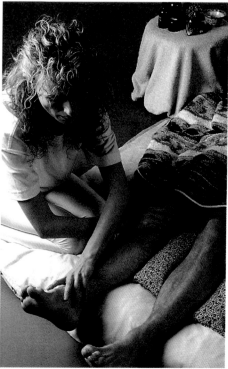

Step 6 – unblocking the knee
Stroke up to the knee and use the pads of the thumbs to work all around the knee cap employing small circular pressures.

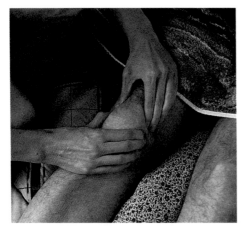

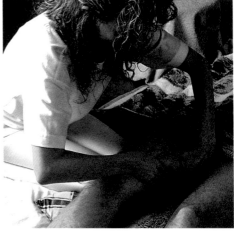

Step 7 – unblocking the thigh
Use firm alternate hand stroking movements working from the top of the knee cap to the lymph glands on the inside of the thigh.

Step 9
Without losing contact, move to the other side of the receiver and lean over to squeeze the muscles of the outer thigh firmly.

Step 10 – connecting the front of the leg
Cover the leg and rest one hand on the hip and the other on the top of the foot to connect the energies.

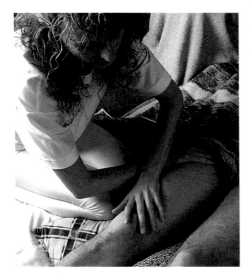

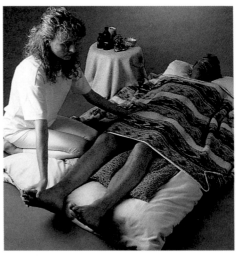

Step 8 – releasing the toxins
With alternate hands pick up, squeeze and bring the muscles of the inner thigh towards you to reduce cellulite and to aid in the elimination of toxins.

Repeat on the other side.

Upper chest, neck and shoulders

Chest

Step 1 – tuning in

Position yourself at the head of the receiver. Place both hands on the front of the shoulders, taking a few deep breaths trying to sense any congestion.

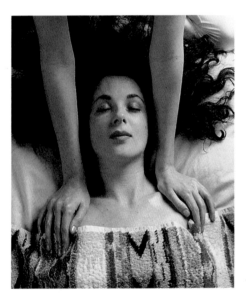

Step 2 – awakening the chest

Place the heels of both hands on the centre of the chest with the fingertips facing towards each other. Stroke from the centre of the chest outwards and downwards towards the lymph glands in the armpits. Repeat this movement.

The upper chest is often an area of congestion and is held tightly in contraction due to the shoulders being held forward. Some people (especially men) experience chest pains which they falsely believe to be indicative of heart problems. A great deal of unresolved emotion may be stored in this area. Since there are many lung pressure points on the upper chest, bronchial problems will also improve.

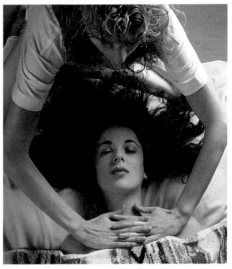

Step 3 – unblocking the lymph

Place both thumbs in the centre of the chest just below the collar bones and press and release

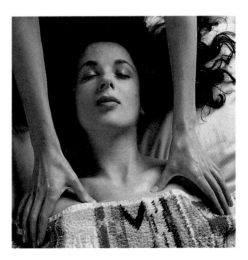

working outwards along the line of the collar bone towards the shoulders. Repeat this movement gently several times.

Step 4 – draining the lymph
With the thumbs in the same position press and drain towards the armpits. Repeat several times.

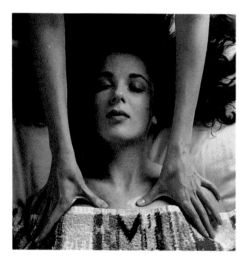

Neck and shoulders

Step 5 – releasing tension at the back and front of the shoulders
Place your hands underneath the receiver's shoulders. Perform large circular movements with the palms of the hands to cover the upper back and the back of the shoulders. This movement is easier if you are working on a couch since you can rest the forearms on the table. Move your hands round to the front of the body to massage the top and front of the shoulders. Use the palms of the hands to make large, circular outward movements until you feel the tightness dissolve.

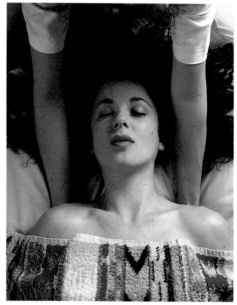

Step 6 – releasing neck tension
Turn the head to one side. Rest one hand on the side of the face and stroke the other hand firmly down the neck and over the shoulder and repeat until the tightness softens.

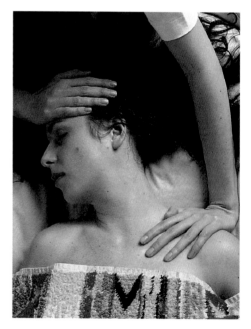

Face and scalp

Now that any lymphatic congestion has been drained from the chest area, we can begin on the face and scalp. It is pointless releasing the lymph in the face if the chest area has not been unblocked first. Aromatherapy treatment of the face and scalp can alleviate headaches and nasal problems such as sinusitis and, in combination with rejuvenative oils, can slow down the ageing process. Stress and tension is reduced and circulation to the head is improved.

Step 1 – drawing energy down

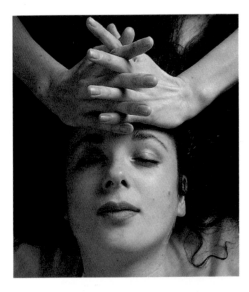

Bring the palms of the hands towards each other, little fingers touching, imagining that they are a cup and rest them gently on the receiver's forehead. Draw healing white light down onto the head with your fingertips. Stroke the healing energy out across the forehead, stroke outwards across the cheeks, across the chin and finally down the neck. Repeat several times.

Step 2 – decongesting the forehead

Place both thumbs in the centre of the forehead just above the eyebrows and work outwards towards the temples. Press firmly and release at about one-inch

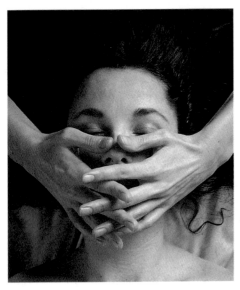

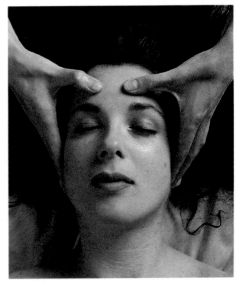

intervals. After your first row bring the thumbs back to the centre of the forehead but move them up slightly. Repeat these rows until you reach the hairline.

Step 3 – decongesting the cheeks and chin

Repeat the technique described in the last step. To decongest the cheeks, start at the top of the cheek bone working down towards the ears in horizontal rows. For the chin commence under the mouth in the centre of the chin working outwards.

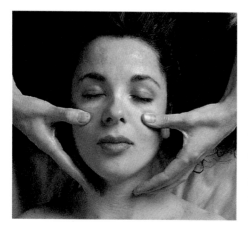

Step 4 – decongesting the brow and nose

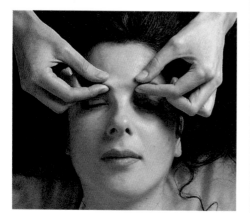

Commencing at the inside of the eyebrows pinch the brow bone. Work outwards until you reach the end of the eyebrow. Repeat several times.

Stroke down the sides of the nose using both thumbs. Repeat several times.

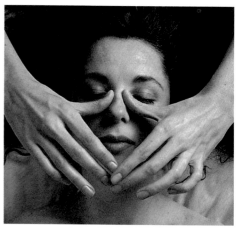

These movements are excellent for the sinuses and catarrh.

Step 5 – awakening and relieving tension in the scalp

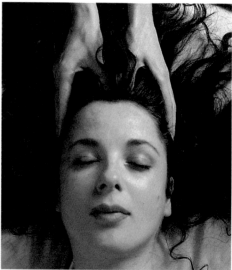

Place the fingers at the back of the skull around the hairline. Firmly and slowly massage the scalp using all the fingers simultaneously. Repeat these movements until the entire scalp has been covered. You should actually feel the scalp moving under your fingertips.

Step 6 – releasing the toxins
Gently run your fingertips through the hair. As you reach the ends of the hair flick the toxins away from the body.
   Finish the sequence by resting the hands gently on the temples. Release them gently.

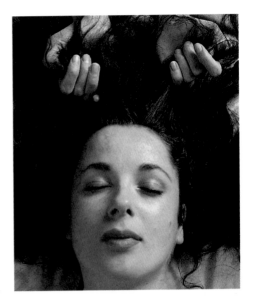

Possible reactions after the aromatherapy treatment

Any reactions occurring as a result of an aromatherapy treatment should be seen as being positive and desirable since this is indicative of the body's innate ability for self-healing. This provides evidence that the essential oils are working. However, do not expect the body to react immediately. Some people will react after one aromatherapy session. Others will require perhaps three or four aromatherapy massages coupled with daily aromatic bathing.

- The receiver will always experience a state of deep relaxation and will sleep much better than before. In a few instances good nights may become disturbed for a while by frequent dreaming – this will occur if an emotional trauma is being released.

- The tone and texture of the skin will improve due to the improved circulation and lymphatic drainage. Occasionally where there is a skin problem such as acne and a detoxifying oil like **juniper** has been used, the skin condition could worsen initially. This is due to the increased activity of the skin as it is encouraged to eliminate more toxins.

- In cases of constipation the essential oils should increase the frequency of bowel movements. Stools will also probably increase in bulk and volume. You will wonder what on earth you have been eating! Stools may occasionally be discoloured and flatulence may increase. This is only temporary and again indicates that the body is casting aside the rubbish.

- In cases of nasal and bronchial problems there may be an increase in the secretion of the mucous membranes of the nose and bronchial tubes.

- The kidneys may secrete more urine particularly if someone has been suffering from fluid retention.

- Sometimes previous illnesses which have been suppressed in the past and which have never truly healed will flare up before they disappear. For instance there may be an attack of cystisis.

- Emotional changes and changes in attitude may also occur.

- In all cases an improved sense of well-being and an increase in vitality will take place.

7

THE SCENTUAL TOUCH FOR PREGNANCY, CHILDBIRTH AND POST-NATAL CARE

With the advance of modern medical science, many people have forgotten that pregnancy and childbirth are the most natural processes in the world. Aromatherapy can be used both to enhance these natural processes and to alleviate minor ailments which may occur. Obviously if symptoms persist then it is always advisable to seek medical attention. When used properly, essential oils are completely safe and harmless and unlike drugs they carry no fear of causing abnormality. Everyone clearly remembers the tragic thalidomide disaster.

Throughout pregnancy babies are very aware of the environment outside the womb and the emotional state of the mother. Since the essential oils that the mother inhales, bathes with and massages into her body are sensed by the baby, aromatherapy can be used very successfully in a variety of ways to ensure that both mother and baby remain in a balanced and healthy state – physically, mentally and spiritually. The essential oils help to induce relaxation, dispel fears and anxieties, relieve the muscular aches caused by the burden of the extra weight and postural changes, improve levels of energy, aid digestion, and improve the circulation to prevent varicose veins and stimulate the lymphatic system to eliminate unwanted fluid and toxins.

I have been privileged to treat many women throughout their pregnancies and they have all enjoyed happy and healthy pregnancies and relatively easy deliveries. As a mother of two young children, Chlöe and Thomas, I also draw from my own experiences. Both my pregnancies were trouble-free and both babies were born after very short labours into birthing pools, using no drugs – not even gas and air. I know I could not have achieved this without my essential oils!

During pregnancy please take care to avoid using the following pure essential oils as they are all said to carry *slight* risks of miscarriage, particularly during the first three months: **basil**, **clary sage**, **fennel**, **hyssop**, **juniper**, **marjoram**, **myrrh**, **rosemary**, **sage** or **thyme**. Also avoid **all** the hazardous oils listed in the appendix. If in doubt, seek advice from a professional aromatherapist.

Always listen to your body and be guided especially by your nose! You will instinctively know which oils to avoid.

When massaging during pregnancy ensure that the movements are very gentle and take particular care when treating the abdomen and lower back. If you are at all worried then simply do not massage these areas.

Essential oils for common ailments in pregnancy

Fluid retention

Oedema is commonly experienced in pregnancy especially in the ankles and wrists. Apply the following blend to tired and swollen ankles.

Dilute in 2 teaspoons of carrier oil:

- 2 drops of **lavender** and 2 drops of **geranium** or

- 4 drops choosing from **cypress**, **lavender** or **geranium**

If breasts are sore at the beginning of pregnancy this formula is equally effective.

Mood swings

Pregnancy produces a flood of conflicting emotions and aromatic baths are wonderful for dispelling the fear of childbirth and motherhood, relieving depression, restoring lack of confidence and uplifting your spirits. Beneficial oils to add to the bath are:

- **Geranium**, **jasmine**, **neroli**, **rose** or **ylang ylang**. Scatter 6 drops into a full bath and feel the tension melt away.

Morning sickness

Nausea is commonly experienced during the early stages of pregnancy and **lavender** or **ginger** will help to keep the stomach calm.

- Either sprinkle 6 drops into your bath or alternatively put 1 drop of **lavender** on the pillow which will also help to induce sleep.

Stretchmarks

Prevention is always better than cure and in order to prevent unsightly stretchmarks massage the abdomen daily. This worked for me! Whilst applying the oil talk calmly and reassuringly to your baby to establish contact. Use one oil or a combination of the following oils:

- **Lavender**, **mandarin**, **neroli** or **tangerine**. Use a maximum of 4 drops in 2 teaspoons of carrier oil.

Tiredness

As the body adjusts to the process of growing a baby, enormous metabolic changes are taking place and it is hardly surprising that extreme tiredness is experienced. To combat fatigue and revive and restore, use one oil or a combination of the following oils:

- **Bergamot**, **grapefruit**, **lavender**, **mandarin** or **tangerine**.

Use up to a maximum of 6 drops in the bath or 4 drops in 2 teaspoons of carrier oil.

Varicose veins

To prevent the arrival of varicose veins caused by the pressure on the legs, aromatherapy massage is a must. Stroke the legs gently working upwards from the ankle to the thigh encouraging circulation and lymphatic drainage.

- Use 4 drops of either **lemon** or **geranium** to 2 teaspoons of massage oil.

Essential oils for the big day

Many midwives are quite willing to allow essential oils in the delivery room. Some enlightened hospitals even have a stock of their own! What a gentle and wonderful way to welcome a baby into the world surrounded by the beautiful aroma of essential oils which he/she is already accustomed to!

Clary sage

Marvellous for pain relief. Almost like administering an anaesthetic! **Clary sage** also facilitates the birth by accelerating mild contractions. It calms, sedates yet uplifts the mother-to-be.

- Dilute 4 drops of **clary sage** into 2 teaspoons of carrier oil and massage into the abdomen or lower back or
- 6 drops in a compress or
- 6 drops in a bath.

Jasmine

An oil for relieving the pain of uterine spasm in the abdomen and back and for facilitating the birth. **Jasmine** also has a powerful sedative effect on the nerves and gives you confidence, support and encouragement to go with the contractions.

- Dilute 4 drops of **jasmine** into 2 teaspoons of carrier oil or
- Use several drops in a diffuser or inhaler.

This oil is expensive but its exquisite perfume justifies the cost.

Lavender

An excellent delivery room oil for purifying the air. It is also very calming and may be used as a compress on the head to pacify the mother. The analgesic properties guarantee its suitability for use as a massage oil on the lower back or abdomen. Lavender also aids in expelling the afterbirth.

- Dilute 4 drops of **lavender** into 2 teaspoons of carrier oil or
- 6 drops as a compress or
- several drops in a burner.

Neroli

This essential oil may be employed to sedate and calm the mother. It will also give the mother-to-be confidence and endurance to go on with what is probably the hardest work she ever does in her life.

- Dilute 4 drops of **neroli** into 2 teaspoons of carrier oil.

The essential oils, which I have described, may also be used in combination with each other. You could prepare the following blend prior to the due date taking care not to inhale too much **clary sage**.

Dilute into 4 teaspoons of carrier oil:

- 3 drops of **lavender**
- 2 drops of **clary sage**
- 1 drop of **jasmine**
- 1 drop of **neroli**

Post-natal oils

Essential oils are absolutely vital after childbirth to prevent and banish post-natal depression and engender calmness, serenity and confidence in the new mother. A relaxed mother leads to a relaxed baby.

Where the birth has been difficult due to a long labour, Caesarean section, use of forceps, vacuum suction, excessive use of drugs etc., it is advisable that the baby be checked by a cranial osteopath, who will gently release any restrictions and compressions in the bones of the cranium. Symptoms such as hyperactivity, excessive screaming or colic, lack of sucking reflex, floppiness and insomnia may present as a result of compression of the cranium at birth. The bones of the cranium are forced up against each other and in severe cases this can cause cot death, brain damage and autism. Disorders such as dyslexia, squints, learning difficulties and personality disorders may also develop. Ideally every baby should be checked.

Breast feeding

Breast milk is, of course, the best possible start for your baby, providing antibodies to disease and reducing the likelihood of allergies. It also is an excellent way of bonding with the newborn. If the milk supply is low then essential oils may be used to promote the flow. To 2 teaspoons of carrier oil add 4 drops of either **fennel**, **geranium**, **jasmine** or **lemongrass**, or alternatively 6 drops of one or a combination of these oils in the bath.

Healing the perineum

To increase the rate of healing, aromatic sitz baths are highly recommended. The lavender will also fight any infections and boost the immune system. Dilute 2 drops of **lavender** and 2 drops of **cypress** into 2 teaspoons of carrier oil and massage into the perineum.

Post-natal depression

To banish the baby blues and balance the emotions and frayed nerves there are a wide variety of oils at your disposal: **bergamot**, **clary sage**, **geranium**, **jasmine**, **mandarin**, **neroli**, **rose**, **rosemary**, **rosewood** or **tangerine**. Choose one oil or a combination from the list above to a maximum of 6 drops in the bath.

Sore nipples

One of the hazards of breast feeding, sore nipples, will benefit from aromatherapy. Wash the nipples thoroughly before each feed so that the baby does not ingest any essential oil. Dilute 1 drop of **rose** or **Roman chamomile** into 1 teaspoon of wheatgerm oil.

8

AROMATHERAPY FOR BABIES AND CHILDREN

Essential oils are particularly valuable and useful when treating babies and children who respond very quickly to this natural method of healing. Their innate powers of self-healing are remarkable since they have not been impaired by years of bad diet, stress, negative thoughts, drugs and pollution. Infants have the ability to throw off their toxins very quickly since their bodies have not been clogged up by toxins accumulated over the years.

Regular use of aromatherapy is an excellent preventative medicine. The child's immune system can be boosted resulting in the avoidance of colds and infections.

Diet is also a major contributory factor in the enjoyment of good health. 'Junk' food seriously impairs a child's capability to eliminate toxic waste. Vaccinations can also be damaging to the immune system preventing it from maturing properly and they also sometimes have serious consequences. If parents took responsibility for their children's diet then vaccinations might not be required. Homoeopathic alternatives are available and I strongly recommend that you find a homoeopathic practitioner for your children.

Even when childhood illnesses do occur, regular use of pure essential oils should very much reduce the length of illnesses, minimise discomfort and prevent secondary infections from occurring.

Roman chamomile in particular is regarded by many as the 'children's oil' since it is low in toxicity and extremely safe and gentle. Other appropriate oils include: **German chamomile**, **lavender**, **mandarin/tangerine**, **rose** or **eucalyptus/tea-tree** (in burners and diffusers).

My preferred carrier oil is sweet almond oil possibly mixed with a small percentage of Evening Primrose oil, jojoba and wheatgerm. The addition of Evening Primrose oil to a blend will significantly improve skin problems.

When bathing a baby or a child always blend the essential oil with a teaspoon of carrier oil. Undiluted essential oil remains on the surface of the water and could be transferred from the baby's hand to the mouth causing injury to the lining of the stomach or to the eyes resulting in permanent damage.

Refer to the following information which shows suitable dosages. Do **not** be tempted to add more essential oil than recommended.

Babies and children

General guidelines

- 5 mls = 1 teaspoon
  10 mls = 1 dessertspoon
  15 mls = 1 tablespoon

Massage

- Babies (0–2 months) – 1 drop per 15 mls carrier oil

- Babies (2–12 months) – 1 drop per 10 mls carrier oil

- Small children (up to 5 years) – 2 drops per 10 mls carrier oil

- Juniors (5–12 years) – 2–3 drops per 10 mls carrier oil

- Adolescents (12 years +) – 3 drops per 10 mls carrier oil

Bath (always dilute in carrier oil)

- Babies (0–12 months) – 1 drop

- Small children (up to 5 years) – 2 drops

- Juniors (5–7 years) – 3 drops

- Juniors (7–12 years) – 4 drops

- Adolescents (12 years +) – 5 drops

Newborn babies

The most suitable essential oils are **Roman chamomile** and **lavender**. I also reach for these two since they are so versatile and will alleviate almost any problem. I have achieved marvellous results with babies.

Colic
A most distressing occurrence, both for baby and parents, characterised by continual screaming which does not disappear even when baby is picked up and cuddled. For speedy relief:

- 1 drop of **Roman chamomile** to 1 tablespoon of carrier oil – gently rub baby's tummy, back and feet *or*

- A compress using 1 drop of **Roman chamomile** applied to the abdomen.

This method usually brings relief without fail. If it is not successful and you are breast feeding look carefully at your diet (see Chapter 9).

Coughs and colds

- 1 drop of **lavender** on some cotton wool placed at the bottom of the crib.

Cradle cap

- 1 drop of **geranium** to 1 tablespoon of carrier oil. Rub *very* gently into the scalp.

Nappy rash
This can be prevented by regular use of essential oils. When washing the baby's bottom dip the cotton

wool into a bowl of warm water into which you have added:

- 1 drop of either **Roman chamomile** or **lavender**

To a 100g jar of zinc and castor oil cream mix in:

- 3 drops of **Roman chamomile** and 3 drops of **lavender**

I personally only use this ointment when the need arises.

Sleep or restlessness

- 1 drop of either **lavender** or **Roman chamomile** – onto a ball of cotton wool at the bottom of the crib or added to a small bowl of warm water placed under the crib.

2–12 months

Coughs and colds
Place a bowl of hot water under the cot or on the radiator into which you have sprinkled:

- 2 drops of either **tea-tree**, **lavender** or **eucalyptus** *or*
- 1 drop of **tea-tree** + 1 drop of **lavender** *or*
- 1 drop of **eucalyptus** + 1 drop of **lavender** *or*
- 1 drop of **eucalyptus** + 1 drop of **tea-tree** *or*
- 1 drop of either **eucalyptus**, **lavender** or **tea-tree** on a cotton wool ball at the foot of the cot *or*
- 1 drop of **lavender** diluted in a carrier oil added to the bath *or*
- 1 drop of **lavender** blended with a dessertspoon of carrier oil and rubbed into the back and chest.

Colic
Rub the baby's tummy in a clockwise direction using:

- 1 drop of **Roman chamomile** mixed in a dessertspoon of carrier oil. If symptoms persist lay a compress on baby's abdomen to which you have added 1 drop of **Roman chamomile.**

Crying or fretfulness

- 2 drops of **Roman chamomile** + 1 drop of **lavender** added to 30 ml carrier oil *or*
- 2 drops of **Roman chamomile** + 1 drop of **geranium** added to 30 ml carrier oil *or*
- 2 drops of **Roman chamomile** + 1 drop of **mandarin** added to 30 ml carrier oil.

Concentrate particularly on stroking the oil into the feet

Skin complaints or allergies
Beware of dairy foods after you have weaned the child as they are usually the culprit. If all parents gave their babies and young children only fruit and vegetables to eat then there would be far fewer health problems!

- 1 drop of **Roman chamomile** or **lavender** in a bath *or*
- 1 drop of **Roman chamomile** per dessertspoon of carrier oil *or*

- 3 drops of **Roman chamomile** + 3 drops of **lavender** added to a 100 g jar of non-perfumed cream.

Sleeping

- 1 drop of **Roman chamomile** or **lavender** into a baby bath or into a bowl of hot water and placed under the cot.

Teething

- 1 drop of **Roman chamomile** blended with a dessertspoon of carrier oil – rub on the outside of the affected side of the face. The Bach Flower Remedy **walnut** is also excellent.

Children

Allergies (e.g. eczema)

Place the child in a bath containing the appropriate dilution of **Roman chamomile** (refer to chart). Massage the affected areas with an oil or non-perfumed lotion with **Roman chamomile** added according to the child's age.

Asthma

- **1–2 years**

1 drop of either **lavender**, **Roman chamomile** or **rose** blended in a dessertspoon of carrier oil.

- **2–5 years**

2 drops of either **lavender**, **neroli**, **Roman chamomile** or **rose** blended in a dessertspoon of carrier oil.

- **5–12 years**

3 drops of either **cypress**, **frankincense**, **lavender**, **neroli**, **Roman chamomile** or **rose** blended in a dessertspoon of carrier oil.

Chamomile, cypress, lavender, neroli and **rose** all relieve spasm and anxiety and **frankincense** slows and deepens the breathing.

Burns

Run the afflicted area under cold water and apply a cold compress using up to 3 drops of essential oil according to age:

- 1 drop of neat **lavender** may be applied to the burn.

Colds or coughs

Massage the back, chest and feet using a blend containing the appropriate number of drops chosen from either **eucalyptus**, **lavender**, **Roman chamomile**, **rosemary** or **tea-tree**.

Constipation

Sitting on the right hand side of your child massage the stomach in a clockwise direction using a blend containing the appropriate number of drops chosen from either **geranium**, **mandarin**, **Roman chamomile** or **rosemary**.

Diarrhoea

Gentle clockwise abdominal massage using a blend containing the appropriate number of drops chosen from either **eucalyptus**, **geranium**, **lavender**, **neroli** or **Roman chamomile**.

Earache

Blend 1 drop of either **lavender** or **Roman chamomile** with a teaspoon of olive oil. Soak cotton wool in this mixture and place in the ear. If pain is severe rub any swollen glands using the appropriate number of drops of **lavender** and **Roman chamomile**.

Fevers

Diluted in carrier oil add to the bath:

- **Eucalyptus** and **lavender** or

- **Tea-tree** and **lavender** or

- **Eucalyptus** and **Roman chamomile**

Cold compresses are also excellent. Up to 3 drops of essential oil may be used. When the compress becomes warm replace it immediately.

Grazes and cuts

Bathe with warm water containing:

- 1 drop of **lavender** plus 1 drop of **tea-tree**. This will calm the child and will not sting as much as proprietary antiseptic.

- 1 drop of neat **lavender** on the plaster will accelerate the healing process.

Headache

Massage and compress. Choose from either **lavender**, **neroli** or **Roman chamomile**.

Infectious diseases

Eucalyptus, **lavender** and **tea-tree** should be burnt in the sick room to prevent the spread of infection.

- **Chickenpox**
  To the bath add **lavender** and **Roman chamomile**.
  To calamine lotion add either **Roman chamomile** and **lavender** or **Roman chamomile** and **tea-tree** and massage.

- **Measles**
  Roman chamomile and **lavender** in oil or calamine lotion.

- **Mumps**
  Blend the appropriate number of drops into a massage oil using either **lavender**, **lemon** or **tea-tree**.

- **Rubella**
  Blend the appropriate number of drops into a massage oil using either **lavender**, **Roman chamomile** or **tea-tree**.

- **Whooping cough**
  Blend the appropriate number of drops for the child's age into a massage oil and rub the chest and add 1 drop to the child's pillow using either **cypress**, **lavender**, **rosemary** or **tea-tree**.

Insomnia

Sprinkle the appropriate number of drops into the child's bedtime bath and add 1 drop to the child's pillow. Choose from either **lavender**, **neroli**, **Roman chamomile** or **rose**.

Lice

As a deterrent add 1 to 2 drops to the final hair rinse. Choose from either **bergamot**, **eucalyptus**, **geranium**, **lavender**, **rosemary** or **tea-tree**.

Stomach pains

Massage with the appropriate number of drops in a clockwise direction. Choose from either **geranium**, **lavender**, **mandarin** or **Roman chamomile**.

Tonsillitis or sore throat
Massage the throat area using the appropriate number of drops into a massage oil using one or a combination of either **lavender, lemon, Roman chamomile** or **tea-tree**.

Veruccae, foot problems or athlete's foot
Apply a massage oil containing one or more of these oils **lavender, lemon** or **tea-tree**.

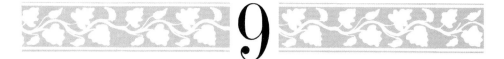

9
MAINTAINING HEALTH

Diet – You are what you eat!

Diet is a very complicated subject in this new age of nutritional awareness. Obviously space does not allow me to explore dietary advice in any great depth but there are many excellent books available for those who wish to pursue it in more detail (see appendix).

As you have probably gathered, I always believe in speaking from my own personal experiences and as a natural health practitioner I have been bombarded over the years by all sorts of diets – vegan, vegetarian, macrobiotic, calorie-controlled and so on, often ending up utterly confused. Finally you have to make your own mind up and choose the diet that is right for you. If you are feeling lethargic, lacking in energy, sluggish, depressed or you are overweight then obviously it is time to change. But whatever you decide to do, do it *slowly*. Dietary changes should *never* be drastic otherwise you may release too many toxins into the bloodstream, feel uncomfortable and positively ill and then will revert back to your former bad habits. Words of encouragement – I have had two children and I am no heavier (in fact I am half a stone lighter) than I was before motherhood. I am certainly more healthy and I do not have much will-power! If I can do it then so can you! But take your time, for rapid detoxification leads to great discomfort.

Diet should not be regarded as a temporary way of life but as a philosophy of living. There is absolutely no point in starving yourself for a week in order to lose weight and then reverting to your former ways and getting fatter than ever. (Does that sound familiar?) The right diet should not only enable you to lose weight but will also, more importantly, allow you to think more clearly and to be filled with far more energy. The need for medical treatment will also be minimised for disease cannot survive in a healthy, clean body. Disease only arises when you have filled your body with so much rubbish that it desperately tries to eliminate the accumulated toxic matter. A good diet does not entail counting calories. It involves eating the right foods.

The essential oils will help you enormously in your daily life. I do implore you to look at your diet. As a therapist I strongly believe in practising what I preach. I would not expect my patients to come for treatments if I was overweight, lacking in energy, negative and unhealthy. If you ever decide to go for treatments, irrespective of the therapy, take a good look at the therapist!

Basically the ideal diet should include a high proportion of fruit, vegetables and salads – about 80 per cent. These foods are regarded to be alkaline. Acid foods such as bread and other starchy foods, meat, cheese, eggs and so on should only form 20 per cent of the diet. It is acids which cause disease – the overproduction of mucus, tension in the nervous system, arthritis, rheumatism, digestive disorders, respiratory ailments and so on.

To start you on the dietary path to health and fitness try to adhere as much as possible to these basic rules:

Do's

- Eat plenty of fresh fruit

- Eat more fresh vegetables (raw if possible)

- Eat more salads

- Chew your food thoroughly and slowly in pleasant surroundings

- Steam or stir-fry your vegetables (if you boil your vegetables then most of the vitamins are left in the water)

- Cook with cold-pressed olive oil

- Have a treat occasionally. You deserve it!

Don'ts

- Don't eat processed foods in cans and packets that contain chemical additives such as colourings and preservatives which are often added to foods during their processing. Additives are harmful and are responsible for much hyperactivity and allergies and may be linked with cancer.

- Don't have too much salt. Replace it with freshly ground pepper, cayenne pepper and herbs. Most processed foods contain salt. Even baby foods contain it so that another salt addict is born. Too much salt leads to high blood pressure, strokes and heart attacks. What children have never had they do not miss.

- Don't have too much sugar which is almost totally lacking in nourishment. It has been linked with heart disease and hardening of the arteries and can cause obesity, tooth decay, mood changes, etc. A healthy diet will provide you with all the sugar you need. Use a little honey if you are desperate.

- Don't eat too much protein in the form of meat especially red meat for it may be linked with heart disease, strokes and cancer. Putrefying waste matter remains in the large intestine for long periods toxifying the body (the average person has 8–12 lbs of rotting waste matter in the colon). Most meat contains chemicals, antibiotics and growth hormones. Try to eat 'low-risk', preferably organically reared meat and more fish.

- Don't have too much protein as in dairy foods which may encourage mucus and a whole host of diseases – arthritis, migraine, allergies, colds, asthma and so on. It is a common assumption for instance that if we don't have dairy foods all our teeth will fall out and our bones will collapse. What a misconception! Calcium from green leafy vegetables and raw nuts is much easier to absorb. Sesame seeds contain huge amounts of calcium so if you are worried sprinkle a few on your food.

- Eating too many fats and oils can result in heart disease. Just use cold-pressed oils or a little real butter.

- Don't drink too much tea and coffee, and don't be taken in by the word 'decaffeinated' which is often no better due to the other chemicals it often contains. A cup of tea or coffee takes about 24 hours to pass through the kidneys and thus places a heavy burden on the body. Reduce your tea and coffee *slowly*. At first try to cut them down by about half. Perhaps even sample a few herb teas – not all of them taste foul, you will be pleasantly surprised! Drink fruit juice and water occasionally.

- Don't mix carbohydrates and protein. Carbohydrates are found in bread, potatoes, cake and sugar. Protein is found in meat, fish, dairy foods and nuts. If you mix them together (as most of us do) an enormous burden is placed upon your digestive system and on your reserves of energy. Digestion takes more energy than anything else – even swimming, cycling and dancing. That's why you feel like sleeping after a heavy meal.

Starch requires alkaline conditions for digestion and protein requires acid conditions. Of course the stomach cannot provide both at the same time. Acid and alkaline neutralise each other.

The system of eating which avoids mixing carbohydrates and protein is often referred to as 'Proper food combining' or the 'Hay Diet'. If it interests you then read more. It's well worth it.

Fasting

Fasting or partial fasting gives your body a spring clean. You clean the outside of your body and possibly spend large amounts of money on it. Why not clean the inside? The energy which is released makes you feel wonderful and cleanses and rebuilds your weak areas.

Water fasting

This involves eating nothing at all and drinking only water. Do not fast for more than three days unless you are under the supervision of a naturopath. The more toxic you are the more headaches and discomfort you will experience. Break the fast with fruit and vegetables, and salads and juices – not with eggs, bacon, mushrooms, tomatoes and fried bread!

Fruit juice fasting

Choose only *one* fruit juice – preferably organic and diluted with water if you wish. If you are very hungry then consume the fruit of your chosen juice. Again do not eat heavy foods immediately.

Fruit fasting
Eat as much as you like of your chosen fruit.

During the fast you will probably feel tired and headachy. This passes and you will feel uplifted, rejuvenated, energy will increase, skin will glow and eyes will look bright.

Exercise and fresh air

Exercise is vital to good health and stimulates the immune system. I am not suggesting that you take up aerobics classes five times a week. Try to take a brisk walk daily. Do it first thing in the morning if possible then you don't have to spend all day thinking about it and making excuses as to why you shouldn't do it.

Exercise and fresh air will make you feel much better. Hippocrates stated 'Eating properly will not by itself keep well a person who does not exercise, for food and exercise being opposite in effect, work together to produce health.'

Skin brushing

Good health is dependent on the skin breathing and eliminating. If this does not occur then the kidneys, liver and lymphatic system will have to compensate and will be overloaded with toxins. Inactivity of the skin is one of the major causes of skin diseases together with poor diet. If the pores of the skin are blocked then the poisons will collect in the skin and lymphatic system. Therefore bathing and brushing the skin will encourage the shedding of dry and dead skin. You will feel and look much more youthful and the battle against cellulite will benefit tremendously.

Skin brushing should ideally be performed at least once a day before your bath or shower. Choose a natural bristle brush, briskly brushing the skin of the whole body. Be gentle at first. Brush in a circular motion, moving from the periphery of the body towards the centre and heart. Where the skin is broken or blemished take extra care. Avoid any sensitive areas such as the face and genitals. If you are pregnant take care on the abdomen. Begin at the feet working *up* both the front and back of the legs. Brush up the buttocks towards the middle of the back. Brush around the abdomen in a circular, clockwise direction following the colon. Finally brush from the hands up the arms and down the chest.

Think positively

Negative thoughts are extremely detrimental to your health and well-being. Negative thoughts attract negative influences. Positive thoughts attract positive influences.

Negative emotions such as fear and panic not only encourage disease but also intensify any underlying illness. The reason that most people die from heart attacks is not the actual attack but the panic that almost invariably accompanies it. The panic further constricts the blood supply to a heart which is already in a precarious condition.

Positive emotions such as love, hope and laughter can interrupt the negative emotions. They protect the body against fear, anger, worry and despair which lead to disease acting like 'blockers'. The positive emotions drive out the negative. It is not possible to entertain two contrary feelings – you can't laugh *and* panic at the same time!

All of us feel depressed at some time in our lives and the result is invariably an illness such as a cold. Next time you feel depressed take yourself to see a funny film.

Thoughts are very powerful so be careful. If you describe others as being a pain in the neck or as a pain in the backside then you probably suffer from either neckache or haemorrhoids! Endeavour to clean up your mind as well as your body.

Bach Flower Remedies are an excellent means for transforming negative thought patterns. Dr Edward Bach formulated his 38 remedies in order to treat the root cause of a problem rather than adopting the traditional orthodox symptomatic approach. These remedies aim to treat states of mind such as fear, depression, envy and indecision which result in disease.

My other book in this series on *Massage* explores the Bach Flower Remedies in greater depth but they must be mentioned here since Bach Flower Remedies and essential oils complement each other so perfectly. They both act on a physical, emotional and spiritual level and they are also derived from plants.

When preparing a blend of essential oils I often add a drop of a flower remedy to increase the effectiveness of the treatment. Alternatively the flower remedies may be taken internally (*not* the essential oils).

Many parallels can be drawn between essential oils and Bach Flower Remedies. There are no rules and you will formulate your own ideas. Use them in a massage or put them in your bath.

Suggested combinations

- **Benzoin** blends with flower remedy **olive** to help alleviate exhaustion of all kinds.

- **Chamomile** blends with flower remedy **impatiens** for anger and irritability.

- **Cypress** blends with flower remedy **walnut** for changes such as menopause, change of job, divorce and so on.

- **Frankincense** blends with **honeysuckle** to let go of the past.

- **Jasmine** blends with **larch** to inspire confidence.

- **Juniper** blends with **crab apple** for those in need of a cleanse.

- **Marjoram** blends with **vervain** to calm and relieve tension.

- **Rose** blends with **holly** where there is jealousy.

Self-aromatherapy

Try to use your aromatherapy every day. Always add essential oils to your bath to stimulate or relax. Add essential oils to your creams and ointments. Sprinkle a couple of drops into your final hair rinse.

Seek a qualified therapist for a professional aromatherapy treatment at least once a month for complete relaxation. (See appendix.)

As Hippocrates said: 'Care for the sick to make them well, care for the healthy to keep them well, and care for yourself.'

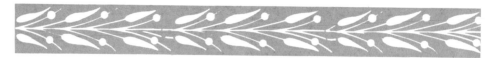

APPENDIX

Hazardous essential oils

The following essential oils should not be used by the lay person, although *some* of them may be used by a professional aromatherapist

Ajowan
Almond (bitter)
Aniseed
Boldo leaf
Buchu
Calamus
Camphor
Cassia
Cinnamon bark
Cinnamon leaf
Clove bud
Clove leaf
Clove stem
Costus
Elecampane
Fennel (bitter)
Horseradish
Jaborandi leaf
Mugwort
Mustard
Origanum
Pennyroyal
Pimento leaf
Pine
Rue
Sassafras
Savin
Savory
Southernwood
Tansy
Thuja
Wintergreen
Wormseed

Pregnancy

As well as the hazardous essential oils the following oils should be avoided by the lay person, to err on the side of safety. A professional aromatherapist may use them.
Basil
Clary sage
Fennel
Hyssop
Juniper
Marjoram
Myrrh
Rosemary
Sage
Thyme

Sensitivity to sunlight

Not to be applied before sunbathing.

Angelica
Bergamot
Grapefruit
Lemon
Lime
Mandarin
Orange

Epilepsy

Fennel
Hyssop
Sage

High blood pressure

Hyssop
Sage
Thyme

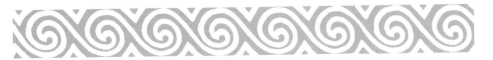

FURTHER READING

Bek L. and Pullar P., *The Seven Levels of Healing*, Rider, London, 1986
Bek L. and Pullar P., *To the Light*, Unwin, London, 1986
Brown D., *Headway Lifeguides: Massage*, Hodder & Stoughton: Sevenoaks, 1993
Chancellor P.M., *Illustrated Handbook of the Bach Flower Remedies*, C.W. Daniel, 1971
Diamond H. and M., *Fit for Life*, Bantam Press, London, 1987
Grant D. and Joice J., *Food Combining for Health*, Thorsons, London, 1984
Kenton L. and S., *Raw Energy*, Century, London, 1984
Valnet Dr J., *The Practice of Aromatherapy*, C.W. Daniel, 1982
Walker Dr N.W., *Diet and Salad*, Norwalk Press, 1971

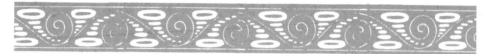

USEFUL ADDRESSES

Beaumont College of Natural Medicine
16 Dittons Road
Eastbourne
East Sussex BN21 1DW
Tel: 0323 724855/641676

For information on professional training courses under the direction of Denise Brown, pure essential oils, base oils, music cassettes, videos, etc.

British and European Osteopathic Association
6 Adelaide Road
Teddington
Middlesex TW11 0AY
Tel: 081 977 8532

The U.K. Homoeopathic Medical Association
243, The Broadway
Southall
Middlesex UB1 1NF

The Society of Homoeopaths
2 Artisan Road
Northampton NN1 4HU
Tel: 0604 21400

I.S.P.A. (International Society of Professional Aromatherapists)
41 Leicester Road
Hinckley
Leicestershire LE10 1LW
Tel: 0455 637987

For a list of fully qualified therapists in your area.

I. F. A. (International Federation of Aromatherapists)
Department of Continuing Education
The Royal Masonic Hospital
Ravenscourt Park
London W6 0TW
Tel: 081 846 8066

For a list of qualified therapists in your area.

Aromatherapy Organisations Council
3 Latymer Close
Braybrooke
Market Harborough
Leicestershire LEI6 8LN

Natural Hygiene Society
Dr K. Sidhwa
3 Harold Grove
Frinton-on-Sea
Essex

The Cranial Osteopathic Association
478 Baker Street
Enfield
Middlesex EN1 3QS
Tel: 081 367 5561

Kirlian Institute
173 Woburn Towers
Broomcroft Avenue
Northolt
UB5 6HV
Tel: 081 841 3458